IMPROVING YOUR RUNNING

IMPROVING YOUR RUNNING

New and Revised Edition

Bill Squires
and
Raymond Krise

The Stephen Greene Press
Lexington, Massachusetts

Copyright © The Stephen Greene Press, Inc., 1982, 1983, 1987

First published in 1987 by The Stephen Greene Press, Inc.
Published simultaneously in Canada by Penguin Books Canada Limited
Distributed by Viking Penguin Inc., 40 West 23rd Street, New York, NY
10010

This work is derived from two earlier books by the authors, *Improving Your Running* (1982) and *Improving Women's Running* (1983).

Line drawings by Laura Hartman Maestro

LIBRARY OF CONGRESS CATALOGING IN PUBLICATION DATA
Squires, Bill.
Improving your running.
Includes index.
1. Running.   2. Running—Training.   I. Krise,
Raymond.   II. Title.
GV1061.S65   1987   796.4′26   86-12074
ISBN 0-8289-0578-9

Printed in the United States of America
by The Murray Printing Company, Westford, Massachusetts
Set in Baskerville
Designed by Beth Tondreau

To my family, former athletes, and coaching associates.
—BS

To Billy Mills, who showed me man could run
six miles fast.
—RK

PREFACE

When we wrote the first edition of *Improving Your Running* in 1981, surveys showed that 30 million Americans were running. Current studies show that 30 million Americans are still running, but they are running fewer miles and fewer races. Many of them do not race at all. Many integrate running with a variety of other athletics. Running remains a part of these athletes' lives, but it means something different to them than it did when they first came to it. It is because of these changes that we have revised this book.

In revising *Improving Your Running,* we've expanded its scope. We've included training programs for people who want to run only for fitness. We've added a program for walkers. We've expanded our discussions of nutrition and exercises for developing the upper body. We have of course continued to offer Coach Squires's training programs for the competitive runner, schedules that have helped readers take 40 minutes or more off their personal records for the marathon.

We strongly suggest that, regardless of what you want from running, you read through the entire book, including all the different training schedules. Our main hope is that you will eventually learn how to coach yourself. The more you understand about the science of training, the better able you eventually will be to customize your own training. The athlete who begins this book wanting definitely to compete, for example, will probably find a day when he or she is injured and needs to train on a schedule that will maintain fitness while letting the injury mend. The competitive runner will also find that he or she can run many races faster if he or she develops upper-body strength beyond what running alone can do. This type of runner will find that advice in Chapter 5 benefits him or her as well as the athlete who runs as a supplement to a more important training program.

Similarly, someone who intends to run only as a supplementary exercise will still learn about how much stress results in how much necessary rest by looking over the programs for the competitive runner.

Frankly, almost no one remains strictly a fitness runner or strictly a racer for all his or her career. Reading the entire book may help you decide just how much of each type of runner you'd like to be.

You will notice that the training schedules give you day-by-day, week-by-week guidance. Look through the schedules and find the week that matches your present fitness level. Do not feel you must run through every week in the whole book. When your body tells you it's absorbing enough mileage, enough wind and rain, enough stress in general, maintain your training or even cut back on it some. When you find that you don't want to run beyond a given stage's level, just keep repeating that stage's final week schedule. Your body will let you know when it's time for you to reach for a higher level of fitness. So will your common sense.

Running is a wonderful experience that makes the body and spirit healthy and strong. The great Czech runner Emil Zátopek once observed that "running is the simplest and most natural movement, like swimming for fish and flying for birds. It is possible to jog till the last day of life." We've tried to make this edition the complete book for the complete runner, to keep you running long enough and happily enough to get enough personal experience to be able to agree with Zátopek.

CONTENTS

Part I

FUNDAMENTALS

1

INTRODUCTION TO RUNNING

It is important that athletes set attainable goals for both themselves and their sport. Given current knowledge of physiology, psychology, and training, it is impossible for anyone to run a sub-3 mile. The athlete who holds that as his or her goal is doomed to frustration, and consequently, may well never realize his or her full potential, which, although certainly less than running a sub-3 mile, might still have equated a world record for the distance.

One of the main reasons why many people begin running is to lose weight and to mold their bodies to a personal model of beauty. The model of beauty varies from one individual to another, and from one culture and historic period to the next; but, basically, people often start running in order to both lose and to redistribute their weight.

THE FIRST STEP IN EXERCISING

The most critical step in exercising, for many people, is finding out first whether or not they should. Strenuous activities such as running and handball are not for everyone. Middle-aged persons may have unsuspected coronary artery disease, and for them the stress of vigorous exercise might be dangerous.

As a general rule, anyone over thirty who is unaccustomed to frequent strenuous exercise should have a thorough checkup before starting an exercise program. The examination should ideally include an exercise stress test, which monitors blood pressure, pulse rate, oxygen consumption, and the heart's electrical activity as the patient exercises. Basically, the standard stress test involves exercising on a treadmill or a bicycle at submaximal intensity and measuring heart rate to find the relationship between the stress of the exercise and the heart. Based on the probable maximal heart rate for someone of your sex and age, the examining physician will impose an exercise intensity that should bring about exhaustion in three to seven minutes. Measuring the respiratory exchange will show whether you are continuing to increase the oxygen consumption in a linear fashion with exercise intensity or whether the exercise has caused your body to demand more oxygen than your body can provide. That's the so-called *breaking point* (which is one determinant of fitness level). The test is valuable for detecting cardiovascular problems that may not show up in an examination of the body at rest. The test also provides data that can serve as guidelines for an individual's exercise program. These tests are given at major medical centers and at many "Y" facilities.

It is best to have an examination within a week or so of the start of your exercise program. It is important that you make a special point of asking the physician for advice concerning the particular activity you intend to begin. A physician who is involved in fitness can be very helpful to anyone interested in exercising.

Remember that a cardiovascular problem detected on examination doesn't necessarily rule out exercise. In fact, exercise may be part of the therapy prescribed. It does mean, however, that the exercise should be undertaken with medical guidance.

MEDICAL INFORMATION

Attention: People with medical disorders.

Medical judgment is a prerequisite for a running program if you have any of the following conditions. Keep in mind that certain *special forms* of exercise may actually be helpful for some disorders, including:

Infectious disease during convalescence of chronic stages
Diabetes controlled by insulin
Recent or active internal bleeding
Kidney disease of any kind
Anemia (hemoglobin less than 10 grams percent)
Any kind of lung disease or disorder
High blood pressure that cannot be lowered beyond 150/90 even
  with medication
Blood vessel disease of the legs
Arthritis (back, leg, feet, ankles)
Convulsive disease not completely controlled by medication

People who have the following disorders must follow their physician's orders regarding *any* form of exercise:

Heart disease or disorders, such as moderate to severe coronary
  heart disease, angina, recent heart attack (within three months),
  severe valvular disease, certain types of congenital disease,
  greatly enlarged heart, and severe irregularities of heartbeat
  that require medication
Uncontrolled diabetes with fluctuating blood sugar levels
Uncontrolled high blood pressure (exceeding 180/110 even with
  medication)
Excessive obesity (greater than 35 pounds excess fat)
Any infectious disease during acute stages

A word to the wise: When in doubt about exercise let your physician have the last word!

THE PLUS OF RUNNING

What does the phrase "chronic effects of exercise" mean? This is the plus factor of running. It is a term used by physiologists, coaches, physical educators, and others to describe the physiological changes that are indexed by exercise over a period of time. The "chronic changes" that take place in a person training for endurance will vary from those that take place in the person training for strength or speed.

Endurance-type exercise generally decreases resting pulse rate; lowers blood pressure, especially diastolic pressure; increases blood volume; increases red blood cells and hemoglobin concentration; improves ability to take in and absorb oxygen; increases muscle tone; and increases the number of blood vessels encircling the heart. The last plus—and this is the reason many people run for fitness—enlarges the arteries so that cholesterol and other fatty deposits are less likely to clog them.

Each of these benefits is a big plus in feeling and looking better. People who begin a running program are amazed to discover that it gives them a sense of well-being and energy that they never had before.

TOOLS OF THE TRADE—WHAT YOU NEED AND WHY

How to Select Running Shoes

Today's running shoe is constantly changing and improving. To choose a good shoe, you must check the sole, the arch, the material, and, of course, the fit.

Since most runners train on asphalt, most running shoes are designed to take the punishment of cement and to protect the foot. A runner places approximately three times the body weight in pressure on the foot. If you run on anything other than sand, the impact goes into the sole of your foot and proceeds to jolt the foot, joints, ankle joint, knee, and hip. It is good to keep that fact in mind when buying shoes for running. It is especially important because a runner makes impact 800 times per mile.

The pressure travels up from the bottom of the foot, so you should first check the sole of a running shoe. A hard sole protects the feet from the shock of running, and it lessens the chance of bone splints. An experienced runner will pick up a shoe and bend it to test its stiffness.

Between the sole and the foot is another protective layer, the cushion. The cushion helps to alleviate stress. The two cushions should have a three-to-one ratio, the top cushion being three times the width of the bottom cushion.

The cushion creates a heel for two reasons: (1) we're all used to wearing a heel, and (2) we use a rocking motion when we run. Running tightens all of the posterior muscles in the body. The motion of the runner is a forward thrust from heel to toe. The longer

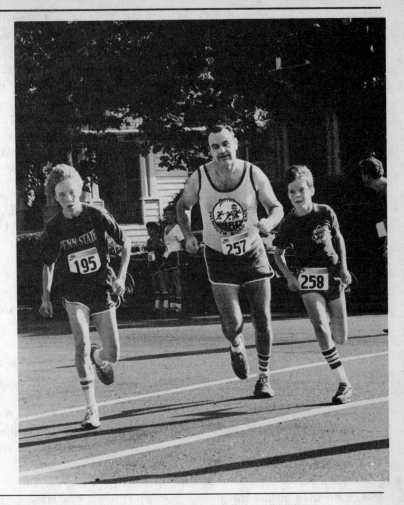

On the road, age makes little or no difference; we're all athletes,
simultaneously competing against and inspiring one another.
(Photograph courtesy of George J. Marcelonis)

the run, the more the runner loses the ability to bring the toe up. It stands to reason, then, that the sole of the running shoe should thicken at the heel.

The heel should be snug, although the heel in a training shoe is different from the heel in a racing shoe, which is cut out for lightness. The arch should be strong and supportive.

Running shoes are made of canvas, nylon, or leather. The material you choose depends on your needs and your body chemistry. Canvas is not very supportive, and it stretches a lot, especially with a lot of sweating. Leather is most supportive, but it allows the least amount of breathing. Nylon is both supportive and air-giving. The best combination is leather for support and nylon for air.

Running shoes are made narrow. You should make sure they feel right on your feet in the store. The best way to try a running shoe is to run in it, but store owners don't want people running out of the store with their shoes, so you should do as much testing in the store as possible.

When you try on a running shoe, it should have forefoot flex and about a thumbnail's space between your toe and the toe of the shoe.

Just as there are material differences in running shoes, there are differences in structure. The sole, for instance, can have a flat surface or a rigid rubber design called "waffles." The protrusions are intended to provide added support, but their benefits are still much debated. Some experts say they are not flexible enough and they upset the runner's balance. Remember, your feet are the best judge.

Training shoes and racing shoes are built differently. Training shoes are heavier than racing shoes. They have higher heels and thicker soles. Trainers are probably your best bet for daily pavement action.

Women's shoes are designed differently from men's shoes. Women's feet are narrower and require a more refined heel. With increased demand, more and more women's models have become available.

Running shoes are made for the forward rocking motion of the foot. The shoe angles downward and can throw a basketball or tennis player off balance. It can also cause sprained ankles in sports that require side to side movements or pivots.

Finally, running purists may not want to admit it, but the multitude of designs, colors, and styles indicate that the cosmetics of the shoe are important. In fact, they sometimes dictate the coordination of an entire spiffy outfit. Maybe they even do a "psych job" for the new or shy athlete.

Clothes

Here are some reminders about the clothes you will need.

Sports briefs. Sports briefs, with high-cut sides, do not show under running shorts and are made with soft-backed elastic to prevent chafing and binding.

Tank top. Cotton mesh tank tops are best. A tank top ideally absorbs perspiration and "breathes" as you run. Remember that light colors, especially white, reflect sunlight. As far as size is concerned, it should be roomy and allow free movement.

Running shorts. Nylon running shorts styled to allow thigh movement are good. Cotton can cause chafing on some people. For others, cotton knits are excellent. It really comes down to an individual's preference.

Running socks. Low-cut cotton peds that absorb moisture and cushion the movement of the foot are best. In winter, regular cotton socks are fine.

Warm-up suits. Only a full-fledged runner needs a warm-up suit. Make an investment, if you feel you must, in a training suit, which is basically a waterproof, lightweight nylon outer suit that is good in rain and snow. Training suits come in colors that are excellent for visibility and also reflect the sunlight.

Wristwatch. It can be inexpensive, but your watch should have a leather or plastic strap and be waterproof. It should have a second hand and should time your run well.

Remember that clothing doesn't have to be the latest fashion. It should be loose and allow the body to breathe. The style is your choice. Just remember that clothes are second to shoes. So put your money into shoes.

Reflective vest. This is a necessary safety item when running at night or in low-visibility weather. The vest is made of material that reflects light from auto headlights and other sources, keeping you safely visible to traffic. Some runners think that putting strips of reflective material on their shoes serves the purpose, but how many drivers keep an eye out for shoes? Look for a vest made of mesh material so you will find it comfortable to wear in all kinds of climates and never be tempted to leave it off when running in the dark.

Sportights. These are tights made of Lycra or a poly-Lycra blend that fit snugly around your legs without impeding circulation or movement and keep you as warm as normal sweatpants but without the bulk or wind resistance. Some athletes prefer them to sweatpants because of their snazzy colors and fit—but some women runners have found that the colors and fit attract unwanted attention and remarks from boorish onlookers.

Hat. When the weather is cold, you'll want a wool cap to help you stay warm. You lose more body heat through your head than through any other portion of your anatomy, so keeping it covered helps keep you warm. If the weather's merely cool, you might find a baseball cap a big help. Its visor offers the additional benefit of keeping sun, rain, snow, sleet, and hail out of your eyes. On a warm rainy day, a simple sun visor will do the same. (In really nasty winter weather, try a combination of wool cap and sun visor—cap over the visor.)

Gloves. A pair of plain cotton painter's gloves will keep your hands warm under most conditions. Cotton thermal hunter's gloves will keep them warm under worse ones. Running with two cotton gloves on each hand will keep your hands warm in the coldest weather in which a person *should* run. A three-glove day means you should stay inside. Gloves from surplus stores are fine. You don't need world-class-runners' signature models.

SELECTING NONESSENTIAL GEAR

Athletes are human. We all want to have gear that we don't really need. Because there is so much more of that type of equipment on the market than there is gear that a runner must have, we won't attempt to outline what to look for in each possible item of equipment. We'll instead suggest three guidelines for helping you to decide if your running would benefit from a new piece of gear you have in mind: (1) Is it fun? (2) Will it contribute to my running and not take away from it? (3) Is there a better, or equally good and less expensive, way to achieve the same result offered by this gear?

Because something is new and/or expensive does not mean that it will be fun to use. Some manufacturers overlook that, along with some consumers. Something might be fun to use, but will also distract you from the real pleasures of running. A personal stereo is an example. A different example is running with weights. Wearing leg weights or holding dumbbells while running will alter your normal running gait. You may become stronger, but your running won't be as much fun as it could be. Running with weight gloves achieves the same effect and also allows you to have fun with your running.

The third guideline should be self-explanatory, but the market now offers some high-tech gear that deserves comment in light of this criterion. There are various electronic pedometers for sale, some of them included in wristwatches, and at least one of them in a pair of "intelligent" microchip shoes. Knowing the exact distance you run would be a training advantage, but all these pedometers depend on being programmed with your stride length—the same as the cheap, old-fashioned pedometer. A runner's stride length changes according to wind velocity, type of terrain, running speed, and degree of athlete fatigue. These devices seem to promise more than they deliver.

The same comment applies to all the personal-computer programs currently available to help guide your training. Not one of them offers more help than you can get by keeping an accurate training diary. (See Chapter 2 to learn how to do that.) You can pick up an adequate diary for five bucks.

If you find yourself attracted to equipment and paraphernalia that help take your attention away from actually getting out and running, you should probably engage in some other sport.

Equipment Alert: Watch Out for Rubberized Clothing

Equipment other than running shoes, clothes, and watch is optional. One word of caution is in order about rubberized suits. Do *not* wear rubberized or plastic clothing while jogging to increase sweating as it will not cause any permanent loss of body weight and can be harmful to your health. Rubberized or plastic clothing can cause your body temperature to rise to a dangerous level because it doesn't allow sweat to evaporate. When sweat cannot evaporate, body temperature increases and causes more sweating, which can lead to excessive dehydration and salt loss, and in turn, to heat stroke or heat exhaustion.

In cool weather, the body gives off heat easily. The body must work harder to cool itself as the weather becomes warmer; there-fore, sweating becomes more profuse. Sweating, in and of itself, does not accomplish anything other than cooling. It does not help you reduce. After a workout, you may find your weight has dropped. The loss, however, is water, not fat, and it will be replaced when you consume water. Sweating does not "clean the pores" as some used to suspect. There is no evidence that sweating is of any value in removing toxic materials from the body, nor does sweating promote fitness. Fitness is developed by exercising the body. Don't interfere with the normal process of regulating the body by using rubberized clothing. You could be making a very serious mistake!

IS RUNNING FOR YOU?

Running is a great sport and can improve your health, but it is not for everyone. No sport is. Neither is vegetarianism. Just because a behavior is generally healthy and fun does not make it a behavior that is right for *you*. If it's not fun, you're not going to stick with it. Give your running (and any other type of new athletics) a trial pe-riod of one full month before deciding finally if you like it. But if you just don't like it, do something else. Don't think there's some-thing wrong with you if you don't like to run. There's only some-thing wrong with you if you don't like to run, and you run anyway.

2

BODY CYCLES: RESPECT THEM!

No one can train hard or race hard all the time. The athlete must understand his or her body's cycles in order to avoid injury and maximize ultimate performance.

There are three different, but interrelated, approaches the athlete can take toward an understanding of his or her personal cycles. The first and most important is keeping the training diary. The second is dividing the year into strength-building and racing seasons; this is a more comprehensive version of the alternating hard and easy training days in the athlete's weekly workout schedule. The third, and most controversial, approach is charting the athlete's physical, mental, and emotional biorhythms. The ideal approach, which no one seems as yet to have perfected, is to blend aspects of these three different methods. The bottom line is that every person is a unique organism. What works for one athlete may cripple the next person. It behooves each of us to discover when we can go hard and when we must back off so we can go hard again another day.

THE ATHLETE'S TRAINING DIARY

You'll note the training schedules in this book provide space for a daily record of comments on each workout. Use the space provided to start your training diary.

Your training diary is a concrete scientific record of what works for you as an athlete, and what does not work for you. The diary should include such data as your waking pulse, your weight, how much sleep you had the night before, how long and how intense a workout you ran, any other exercises you did during the day, peculiar weather and/or terrain conditions, any medication or other drugs (e.g., coffee) you ingested, your emotional attitude, and any aches and pains (no matter how apparently inconsequential) you're experiencing. If you keep a faithful and accurate daily diary, you will have an invaluable means of determining your personal athletic patterns. You will also have an invaluable source of information for any medical practitioner you may have to consult if you become injured.

It may be harder to start keeping a training diary than it was to start the running program in the first place. The athlete sees almost immediate beneficial results from running, but it takes months for the value of the training diary to become manifest. Keeping a trainning diary will also consolidate your commitment to serious training. It will make you feel like a scientific athlete, and that feeling will translate into your becoming even more scientific in your running.

TRAINING'S SEASONAL CYCLES

The year should be divided into two types of season: (1) the off-season base-building cycle, and (2) the on-season energy-expending cycle.

This does not mean the athlete should divide the year into one six-month base-building cycle and one six-month energy-expending cycle. For one thing, you won't be able to hold a racing peak for six months, unless you're Bill Rodgers. For another, most likely you'll have two or three separate seasons during the year in which you'll want to be sharp, and these seasons will probably fall a few months away from each other. For example, runners in New England normally use the months from December to February, inclusive, as an off-season, base-building cycle. The goal during this period is to run 10–15 miles per week more than during the racing season. The athlete should run comfortably during this time. It is not a time of intensive quality workouts. He or she might do one hill session and

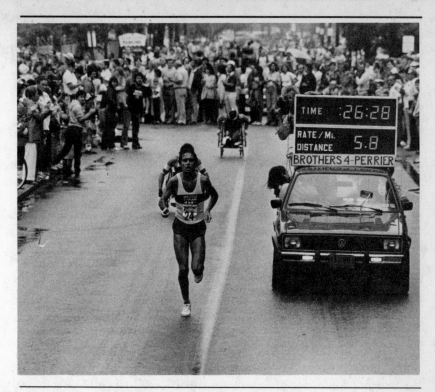

Not even a champion such as Alberto Salazar runs at this kind of pace every day, or his body would break down; learn when to have hard workouts and when to have easy ones. (Photograph courtesy of George J. Marcelonis)

one session of pick-ups (six pick-ups held for 30–60 seconds with a 4:30 or 4-minute rest interval between each) per week. The athlete should also race approximately once a month during the off-season, but should make no effort to peak for the races. Instead, he or she should treat the off-season competition as a means of measuring his or her basal improvement, an index of his or her natural talent.

In New England, runners also use the months of June and July as an off-season time to build up basic strength. The other months, we race. You will notice that our racing cycles in New England come in the spring and the fall, which is when our area has the best weather for racing. Your own geographical area may well be different from ours; consequently, you'll want to time your cycles differently.

Racing tradition also has some influence on when you'll want to build and when you'll want to race. New England runners would still peak for the Boston Marathon if it were held on the hottest day of the year, as it occasionally is. July 4th in Atlanta, Georgia, is hardly the most ideal climatic day on which to run a hard race, but Georgia runners are still going to want to be sharp for the Peachtree 10K. Make your racing plans a year ahead of time, and schedule your off-season and racing-season cycles accordingly.

Being in a racing-season cycle does not mean the athlete is competing several times a week, or even once a week, every week. It requires both significant natural talent (about which you can do absolutely nothing—your genes either gave it to you or they didn't) and many years of careful training before a runner can compete effectively this often. Some of the best-known world-class athletes *never* attain such a level, or even try to attain it. Regardless of his or her level of talent and training, the serious athlete always prefers quality over quantity. One great race is worth myriad mediocre performances as far as a true athlete is concerned.

The serious athlete is therefore advised to take his or her racing-season cycle in three-week periods, meaning he or she races once every three weeks. (In New England, that means the athlete races four times during the twelve-week period of the March-to-May racing season.) Following this recommended cycle, the athlete gets in two and one-half weeks of hard, quality training, takes two to three days to "tone down" and rest for the big race, races, then takes two to three days after the race to build back up to high-quality training. The rule of thumb concerning the two to three days both before and after a race is to "go back up the way you came down." That means you should follow your resting schedule in reverse during the days after the race. For example, if you ran 3 very easy miles the day before the race, you don't run 3 medium-hard miles the day after it—you run the same 3 easy miles.

Results in this program will be apparent after six weeks of racing, because these cycles emphasize *gradual* adaptation to the mental and physical stresses of high-performance running. If the athlete is already serious about training, he or she will discover that the mind adapts much more quickly than the body to the requisite stresses. Remember: "the spirit is willing, but the flesh is weak." No matter how gung-ho your mental attitude, you *must* give your body time to make its physiological adaptations. Nobody races well when injured.

BIORHYTHMS: YOUR PERSONAL, MENTAL, PHYSICAL, AND EMOTIONAL CYCLES

The athlete may want to consider keeping track of his or her personal biorhythms, especially when trying to select key races for which to peak. The athlete should also be aware that, as far as medical science is concerned, biorhythm theory has been neither conclusively validated nor discredited. As with any other training aid, what works for Athlete A may injure Athlete B. Still, no discussion of the relationship between the body's cycles and athletic training should overlook mention of biorhythms.

Fundamental biorhythm theory is simple and plausible: There are times when the intellect, the emotions, and the body are "up" and there are times when they are "down." Everyone has experienced "good days" and "bad days," times when we were profoundly surprised with our behavior either favorably (good days) or disastrously (bad days). The theory holds there are three distinct cycles to the rhythms governing intellect, emotion, and physical performance. *In theory,* the physical cycle takes twenty-three days (eleven days "up," ten days "down," and two days when the rhythm is crossing from down to up, or from up to down—called "critical days"), the emotional cycle takes twenty-eight days (thirteen days "up," thirteen days "down," and two "critical days"), and the intellectual cycle takes thirty-three days (sixteen days "up," fifteen days "down," and two "critical days"). It should be emphasized that, according to empirical observation, the "up" days of the cycles do not necessarily mean days on which you'll inevitably be a superstar, any more than the "down" days of the cycles doom you to incapacity. Experience indicates that the more "up" the cycle, the more resilient or flexible the mental, emotional, or physical capabilities of the person will be. The more "down" the cycle, the less flexible or resilient will be the capabilities. For example, even at the peak of one's emotional cycle, he or she will still be distraught to hear of the death of a close friend, but will be better able to cope with and accept the tragedy than if the news had come during a "down" portion of the cycle.

It's interesting to note that it is only in the emotional cycle that the "up" and "down" segments of the sine curve mirror each other. In the physical cycle, there are two days when the curve is at top-dead-center and only one day when it is down at absolute bottom. In the intellectual cycle, on the other hand, there is only one day of peaking on the up-curve, and two days down in the pits on the down-curve. This may say something about the exigencies of human evolution, when physical prowess was more imperative to survival than was intellect.

A few well-publicized studies of the relationship between biorhythm theory and athletic performance have presented data the researchers interpreted as "debunking" biorhythm theory. This leads us to a discussion of how the athlete can use biorhythms to his or her advantage. The studies referred to charted the physical biorhythm of top athletes, then compared their actual performance in sport to what their biorhythm seemed to predict would be their performance. The studies concluded there was no correlation between athletic performance and alleged biorhythm. For example, one such study cited Bill Rodgers in the 1979 Boston Marathon, in which he set a new American record while theoretically down in the physical biorhythm pits. The problem with such studies is that it is hogwash to focus only on the *physical* biorhythm. The long-distance runner runs with his or her emotions at least as much as with his or her legs. The researchers neglected the fact that Rodgers's emotional biorhythm was at top-dead-center that day in Boston. Billy, and others in his league, is so physically gifted that he can run world-class times even in the physical biorhythm dumps provided he is "up" for the race. You can, too.

In short, the athlete should pay attention to both physical and emotional peaks and valleys. If there is a race you really want to run but the 'rhythms are low, that doesn't mean you should not run the race. It only means you should make contingency plans to accommodate your relative lack of spunk on that date.

Your training diary will ultimately reveal your own personal up-and-down pattern. It does not, frankly, seem reasonable to presume all people are locked into precise twenty-three-, twenty-eight-, and thirty-three-day cycles. If you would like to try plotting your biorhythms according to the theory and correlating them with your training, though, Casio makes a handy combination calculator-and-biorhythm computer called a Biolater that is inexpensive and widely available.

3
DIET AND NUTRITION

HOW RUNNING AND DIET AFFECT EACH OTHER

It may sound illogical, but the more you exercise, the less you will probably want to eat. This is particularly true within the first 15 minutes after the end of your workout. The sensation of hunger is not a function of how much food is in your stomach. Instead, it is a function of your blood-sugar levels. The more sugar in your blood-stream, the less hungry you feel. That is why drinking a cup of coffee or taking a "diet" pill depresses your appetite. The caffeine in these substances causes the body to secrete adrenalin, which makes you feel less hungry. Prolonged exercise does the same thing, with none of the side-effects of drugs. The adrenalin released by exercise raises your blood-sugar level for 15 minutes or so after the cessation of work.

Not only does exercise actually depress the appetite, it raises your metabolic level both during and after the workout. You are not only burning off calories while you run, you are also burning them off at a higher rate than normal for some time *after* you're done running. The longer your workout (in terms of time, not necessarily in terms of distance), the longer your metabolic rate will be elevated.

Running helps burn off excess calories, and, consequently, excess pounds. Running depresses the appetite. Running also seems to make the body use the fuel (food) it takes in more efficiently. In other words, a fit person can perform a given amount of work using less food than an unfit person. This means that runners want to eat less food, relative to the amount of work they are performing, than their sedentary counterparts.

It is human nature to resist behavior one finds unpleasant. Both dieting and simultaneously beginning a jogging program are very unpleasant experiences. Dieting entails additional physical and emotional stress on the human organism. Any attempt to change one's habits creates a stress on the individual, even if the attempted change is both pleasurable and beneficial. (Falling in love is an example of a positive form of stress; it usually results in as many sleepless nights as giving up smoking.) Starting a new exercise program also brings stress into a person's life. An exercise program— such as the running schedules contained in this book—demands that the body have an abundant supply of *easily burned* fuel. Fat is a fuel very hard for the body to burn (metabolize). That is precisely why it is fat: it's nature's nutritional "savings account," stored away for the rainy (and, in our society, improbable) day when you find yourself literally starving. The person who tries to exercise on fat stores alone is asking for trouble, and, ultimately, discouragement.

In practical terms, don't make a conscious effort to cut back on your caloric intake if you want to lose weight. Just go out and run instead. Regular exercise will reduce the amount of food you want to eat, lower your appetite, and lessen the amount of fat your body *wants*.

Although we suggest you do not try to cut back on your caloric intake, you would be wise to alter the food sources from which you derive those calories. This is yet another phenomenon of which your body would naturally apprise you, but there is no harm in your anticipating it. Reduce the amount of fat and protein in your diet, and raise the amount of carbohydrates. The normal American's diet ratio of these food sources is 15 percent protein, 40 percent fat, and 45 percent carbohydrate. Try shifting to 15 percent protein, 30 percent fat, and 55 percent carbohydrate. You might eventually find you're eating a much higher percentage of your diet as carbohydrate than 55 percent, but use these figures as rough guidelines for starting out. By eating less fat and more carbohydrate, you will give yourself the fuel to continue with your running and will give your body less craving to add fat.

NUTRIENTS AND FOOD SOURCES: WE ARE WHAT WE EAT

The body needs *carbohydrates* to supply energy, prevent ketosis, conserve certain minerals, furnish heat, and save proteins for building and regulating cells. Carbohydrates consist basically of sugars and starches. Food sources are fruit, most vegetables, flour, cereals, bread, potatoes, honey, dried beans and peas, peanut butter, rice, and corn.

Proteins are essential for building, repairing, and regulating the function of the body's cells. They are found in meat, fish, poultry, eggs, cheese, milk, nuts, dried peas and beans, bread, cereals, and vegetables. Although protein has an energy-giving quality, its true functions are growth and repair.

Fats are a secondary but important source of energy. A stored form of energy that the body does not utilize immediately, fats are contained in butter, margarine, cream, oils, meat, whole milk, peanuts, nuts, and avocados.

Remember: Carbohydrates, proteins, and fats are energy-yielding substances. Remember, too, that vitamins, minerals, and water do not yield energy but are necessary to proper body functioning.

Vitamins are essential to life, and they directly or indirectly influence all metabolic processes in our bodies. There are water-soluble vitamins (B complex and C), excess amounts of which the body can excrete in the urine, and fat-soluble vitamins (A, D, K, and E), which are stored in the fat cells. A daily intake of vitamins in excess of the recommended dietary allowance may be potentially dangerous because of the absence of excretory pathways.

Sources of *fat-soluble vitamins* include:

Vitamin A: Cheese, green and yellow vegetables, butter, eggs, milk, fish, and liver. Converted from carotene in vegetables by the liver.
Vitamin D: Fatty fish, eggs, liver, butter, fortified milk. Produced in skin on exposure to ultraviolet rays in sunlight. Essential for body metabolism of calcium and phosphorus.
Vitamin E: Vegetable oils and wheat germ.
Vitamin K: Eggs, liver, cabbage, spinach, and tomatoes.

What does a fat cell do for the body? It provides fuel, or energy. Of course, fuel also comes from other sources, such as *glucose* (what sugars and starches are converted into), which is the most popular "quick service" fuel. *Glycogen* is the short-storage form of starches that converts easily to glucose for emergency energy needs. Fat is the long-term storage form of energy, but it too can be mobilized— changed into glucose or used as fatty acids—for energy when needed.

The body's first choice of fuel is usually glucose, followed by glycogen and then fat. The fat deposits are stored under the skin and around the heart, liver, pancreas and even between muscle fibers until the body needs them, for example, between meals when the glucose and glycogen have been used up. Chances are good that fat reserves will never be called up because the body is constantly taking in new fuel. Anywhere from 3000 to 4000 calories worth a day is the average food intake for many adults. A calorie is a unit of measurement used to describe how much energy will be produced by the food you eat after it has been digested for use by the body. One pound of fat is equal to 3500 calories.

Now, if you eat food containing 3000 calories and you only use 2500 worth that same day, you'll have 500 calories worth of food energy to spare. Any extra food energy not used immediately is stored as fat. If you overeat this way for seven days, you'll gain a pound.

How does the body burn off all those calories?

Well, you're burning off some of them even when you're resting. Your body needs energy twenty-four hours a day to keep its temperature at 98.6°F, and you've got to have energy to keep those vital organs functioning—your heart always beats, you breathe, you blink, you move your muscles.

The rate at which you use energy just to keep your body going when you're resting is called your *basal metabolic rate*, or BMR, for short. Basal metabolism, of course, varies with each individual because internal energy needs are different—due to size, age, and other variables. Normal body functioning accounts for part of your energy needs. You can change your BMR and the number of calories you need by changing your body's activities. If you want to burn up more calories, you're going to increase your external activities (calorie needs over and beyond the BMR) with exercise.

Of course, the body's a little more complex than that. Sometimes your hormone balance alters and causes your BMR to change, because it's regulated by the hormone thyroxin. Or sometimes you have too much or too little insulin, which metabolizes glucose, and so your calorie needs change. Don't forget, the body is terribly efficient. It doesn't waste anything. It even converts some food elements, such as protein, into glucose or other goodies the body needs for energy and repair work before it resorts to using up fat cells. How long we can stay around depends, in part, on what we do or do not eat daily.

Sources of *water-soluble vitamins* are as follows:

Thiamin (B): Meat, whole grains, liver, yeast, nuts, eggs, beans, soybeans, and potatoes. Necessary for carbohydrate metabolism and combatting nervousness and fatigue.

Riboflavin (B): Milk, cheese, liver, beef, eggs, and fish. Essential for metabolism in all cells.

Niacin: Bran, eggs, yeast, liver, kidney, fish, whole wheat, and tomatoes. Necessary for growth and metabolism.

B$_{12}$: Meat, liver, eggs, milk, and yeast. Needed for production of red blood cells and growth.

Ascorbic acid (C): Citrus fruits, cabbage, tomatoes, potatoes, and leafy vegetables. Needed for cellular metabolism and energy.

Minerals are important components of bone and tissue and are essential to the regulatory processes of the body. Those known to be needed by the body are calcium, chlorine, cobalt, copper, fluorine, iron, iodine, magnesium, manganese, phosphorus, potassium, sodium, sulfur, and zinc. Most minerals are found in fats, oils, flour, cereals, breads, potatoes, sugar, liver, beans, peas, and peanut butter. Two or more glasses of water each day also provide some minerals. Sources are:

Calcium: Milk, dried skim milk, ice milk (dessert), cheese, dark-green leafy vegetables, and whole grain products

Iron: Dried beans and peas, liver, whole grain or enriched breads, cereals, dark-green leafy vegetables, eggs, less expensive meats, potatoes, sweet potatoes, and prunes

Potassium: Meat, fish, bananas, baked potatoes, vegetables, and fruit. Very important to replacement of fluids lost through perspiration.

Phosphorus: Meat, liver, bacon, whole grains, cornstarch. Necessary for enzyme system to release energy needed for metabolic action.

Iodine: Iodized salt. Important for proper metabolism.

Water is excreted from the body in the urine, in the feces, in perspiration, and through evaporation from the lungs during exhalation. Food intake accounts for about two quarts of the approximate water requirement of three quarts a day. The additional amount should be obtained by drinking fluids. Water is important because it distributes heat throughout the body, facilitates the chemical reactions of metabolism, and promotes digestion. If you are moderately active, you need three quarts per day. This will be your guideline.

WHAT NOT TO EAT

The handiest diet rule for a runner to follow is to try to choose from a high-carbohydrate menu while also indulging in whatever foods he or she truly craves. However, it takes some practice to learn what cravings result from nutritional need and which ones result from force of self-indulgent habit. Therefore, we offer this basic list of types of food to avoid. Only rarely do these goodies contribute to good nutrition, but we frequently yearn for them anyway. We've learned to love their taste.

Avoid: dairy products with cream in them (including whole milk and most cheeses), fried foods, red meats, sausage, duck, goose, shrimp, caviar, sugar, lard, most pastries and other baked goods, olive oil, chocolate.

A simple way to remember this list is try to eat foods low on the food chain and avoid those high on the food chain. This also means staying away from processed foods. In general, the closer a food is to having just grown out of the ground, the more nutritious it is. The heat of cooking destroys nutrients—so do most other forms of food processing, such as refining, aging, or peeling. This sort of nutritional consideration leads many endurance athletes to become vegetarians. You individually may neither need nor want to give up animal foods. We're just urging you to be aware of the freshness and nutritional value of your diet.

CLIPPING CALORIES

Since many of us enjoy eating "junk" foods—or at least foods that are delicious and high in calories—and, at the same time, want to watch our weight, we face an obvious problem. Is it a matter of "either/or"? Maybe not! If we are moderate in both our eating habits and our exercise, we should be able to control our weight. Basically this unique way of thinking equates a doughnut with a thirty-minute walk and a hamburger with a forty-minute jog. Equating exercise and food can be very helpful, but it takes into account only the caloric value of foods, not their nutritional value. Keep in mind that for energy and total health we must have a nutritionally well-balanced diet.

For those of you who like snacks but are concerned with calories, the following chart tells how many minutes of jogging are necessary to burn off those extra calories.

Food	Amount	Calories	Walking	Jogging
Spaghetti & meatballs	2 cups	345	69	35
Chicken TV dinner	10 oz.	542	104	54
Pizza, 14-inch	⅛	185	36	19
Hamburger on bun	4 oz.	375	75	38
Peanut butter and jelly sandwich	2 T.	290	55	29
Tuna, water pack	3½ oz.	127	24	13
Pancake with butter and 1 T. syrup		240	46	24
Cheese omelet	1 egg	219	43	22
Yogurt, plain	1 cup	150	29	15
Soybeans, cooked	2 oz.	80	16	8
Brown rice, cooked	1 cup	178	34	18

Food	Amount	Calories	Walking	Jogging
Dinner roll	1 avg.	90	18	9
Apple	1 med.	80	16	8
Strawberries	10 fresh	37	7	4
Peanuts, dry roasted	2 oz.	320	60	32
Popcorn, plain	1 cup	25	5	2
Potato chips	15	172	34	17
Ice cream	1 cup	270	54	27
Cheesecake, 9-inch	$\frac{1}{12}$	300	60	30
Chocolate chip cookie	2 med.	100	20	10
Chocolate	1 oz.	152	29	15
"Ritz" crackers	4	68	13	7
Orange juice	4 oz.	60	12	6
Cola	12 oz.	155	30	16
Wine, dry	4 oz.	98	20	10
Beer	8 oz.	114	23	12

Attention pizza-lovers: Recently, a laboratory test reported that a thirteen-ounce frozen pizza supplies an adult with 66 to 75 percent of the Recommended Daily Requirement (RDR) of protein, up to 127 percent of the

*calcium, 55 percent of the iron, 50–100 percent of the thiamin, 66 percent
of the riboflavin, 70 percent of the niacin, and 900 to 1150 calories. You
figure out how much jogging you'll have to do to burn all that off!*

FOOD FACTS FOR RUNNERS

If you are running to lose weight, you should know that exercise
helps in weight reduction, but dietary habits are the most important
factor. Therefore, avoid or use sparingly fried foods, fatty meat (cut
all visible fat from meat) and fish, gravies and cream sauce, regular
carbonated beverages and alcoholic beverages, rich desserts and pastries, cookies, cakes, pies, and concentrated sweets (candy, jelly, jam,
honey, molasses, and sugar).

Carbonated drinks should be eliminated during the season because they increase the amount of carbon dioxide in the blood.

Digestion facts to keep in mind are:

1. It is unwise to exercise within two hours of a meal, for it takes
    two hours for food to pass through the stomach.
2. Fat and protein are slow (three to five hours) in getting out of
    the stomach and into the digestive tract.
3. Protein residue is given off through the kidneys. During exer-
    cise, an athlete's kidneys are shut down and wastes aren't ex-
    creted. Therefore, runners eat protein sparingly before a race.
4. If you don't eat, you may feel sluggish because your body
    could be running short on energy.
5. An athlete should have extra liquids before an event because
    he or she will be sweating so much. Adding extra salt to food
    will prevent too much fluid loss.
6. If you eat right before exercising, your blood is diverted to all
    the exercised parts of the body from the digestive tract and
    kidneys where it would normally aid in digestion. Result: your
    food sits at the bottom of your stomach.

NUTRITION TIPS FOR MASTERS

Persons over the *age of 50* need fewer calories because they are less
active. They do need as much protein as healthy young adults, plus
supplements of iron and vitamin B_{12} to prevent anemia, calcium for

bones and teeth, and especially fiber such as bran for healthy intestines. All masters should plan to avoid "junk" foods.

DO YOU NEED TO TAKE SUPPLEMENTS?

Probably not. Unless you are a special medical case, a normal, balanced diet will give you all the nourishment and vitamins you need as an athlete.

These past few years have seen a change in attitudes toward health-care in our society. Growing numbers of people attempt to be their own practitioners. While the trend toward preventing illness instead of reacting to it after the fact is certainly praiseworthy, the trend toward rejecting medical data in favor of the sales pitches in "health food" stores must be deplored. One major problem arising from this trend is the belief that megadoses of vitamins are good for one. In some instances, megadoses of vitamins are harmful only to one's fiscal health; in others, vitamin overdose may cause harm.

There is one type of diet with which it would be wise to take a vitamin supplement: vegetarianism. A vegetarian is smart to take a vitamin B–complex supplement. (By the way, we've noticed that some people who eat fish and fowl consider themselves "vegetarians." We don't want to get into a lexicographic argument here, but if you are this kind of "vegetarian," you don't need to take a B-complex supplement to be on the safe side. *Your* kind of "vegetables" contain every class of B vitamin known.)

The average woman might consider taking an iron supplement. One study of distance runners, conducted in 1981, found that 82 percent of the women tested (and 29 percent of the men) were at risk of iron deficiency. The athlete is urged to consult a physician or other reputable health professional for an assessment of her own particular plasma ferritin concentrations before starting on iron supplements.

Caffeine, although of no nutritional value in itself, is a dietary supplement the athlete may consider using occasionally. (Please be sure to read the discussion of the physiological effects of caffeine in Stage 4R of the training schedules.) Caffeine, contained in coffee and many teas, has been shown to help improve performance in some endurance athletes. It is a supplement that should be used sparingly, and with a sound knowledge of its effects on the body in general, and on the individual in particular.

PRERACE MEAL: IT'S IMPORTANT!

Eat your prerace meal no later than three hours before the competition; ideally, you will have finished eating it long before then. As long as you select from the types of foods listed below, your meal will be digested before the gun goes off.

In the hour before the race, you might consider drinking a strong cup of coffee. The caffeine in the coffee will help you burn your body's fuel more efficiently. It does this by releasing free fatty acids into the bloodstream. The body would rather burn free fatty acids than glycogen, but it would rather burn glycogen than it would normal fat. By eating a diet high in carbohydrates as part of your normal training, you will have built up glycogen stores. Drinking the caffeine helps you save those stores for when you really need them.

Something to avoid on race day is food with sugar. This is especially true in the hour before your event. Eating sugared foods at that time will have the opposite practical effect of drinking coffee: It will accelerate the rate at which you burn up glycogen.

Instead of eating a thick, juicy steak before a race, try spaghetti with tomato sauce topping, waffles, pancakes, macaroni, bread, crackers, rice, fruit juice, honey, baked or boiled potatoes, fruits, cereals, or apple sauce. A limited intake of coffee or tea with the meal is fine. Many coaches and trainers do wonders in healing the injured, but they don't know much about nutrition. To be healthy and ready for competition one must have enough pep to do a day's work effectively, be reasonably certain of surviving a physical emergency, and have sufficient reserve energy to enjoy leisure time.

You want to get maximum results from your food intake during a race. Here is a sample menu that will work well for most people.

IDEAL MEALS BEFORE RACING

Breakfast

Choose from:

Cereal: corn flakes, rice cereal, cooked cereal, etc.
Bread: toast, rolls, with jam or syrup or honey
Fruit: canned peaches
Cooked items: pancakes with syrup, waffles with syrup
Tea or water

Lunch or Dinner

Choose from:

Spaghetti with tomato sauce, macaroni, or plain pizza
Crackers or bread
Tea or water

After Meet Meal

Choose from:

Sandwiches, cheese, chicken, turkey
Soup: tomato
Cooked food: meat (lean), fish, potatoes (boiled, mashed), corn,
   beets, rice
Bread or crackers
Juice: apple, orange
Fruit: canned or fresh
Tea, milk, water, or yogurt

During the two days following a race, eat plenty of protein.

THE ATHLETE'S DIET AND DENTAL CARE

A high-carbohydrate diet poses a danger to dental care, and you should be aware of it. Carbohydrates are an efficient athletic fuel because they easily break down into sugars that the cardiovascular system transports to the muscles for work. The problem is that carbohydrates break down so readily into sugars that the process begins right in your mouth. Even though you avoid sugar (and, we hope, all other concentrated sweeteners, no matter how raw and "natural") in your diet, you are still washing your teeth in sugar by consuming a high-carbohydrate diet. Sugar is sugar, whether refined white or broken-down carbohydrate, and its effect on your teeth is the same. It damages them.

We strongly recommend that you consume a high-carbohydrate

diet; but we also urge you to brush your teeth right after dining. If you wait more than 15 minutes between eating and brushing, the damage will be done, and brushing may sweeten your breath and please your toothpaste company, but it won't help to protect your teeth.

4

BECOMING STRONG AND HEALTHY

YOUR BODY AND YOUR RUNNING

A realistic assessment of your current physical strengths and weaknesses will help you determine what sort of exercises you need to supplement your present strength, and, just, as if not more important, what sort of races you should run.

It is possible to reach such determinations through the relatively simple procedure of a muscle biopsy, which can also be combined with a comprehensive stress test to measure such performance factors as maximal oxygen volume uptake and maximal pulse rate. The East Germans have become particularly scientific in this regard, going so far as to measure levels of lactic acid and percentage of red blood cells and high-density lipoproteins in an athlete's system within seconds after he or she completes a workout. The East Germans also carefully monitor the genetic makeup of children to determine athletic potential.

There is a simpler, and practically equally effective, means to gather such data: Watch yourself run. Keep track of your times while competing in events of different length. If you have trouble maintaining proper arm carriage, for instance, you need to work out to strengthen your arm muscles. If you're afflicted by side stitches, you need to do more bent-knee sit-ups (and try doing sit-ups "side-ways," too—a few while lying on each side—to strengthen your girdle muscles all the way around). If you finish in the top 10 habitually in 10-milers but get left in the dust when the gun goes off for a 10K, there's a great future for you in *long*-distance running, but you're not a sprinter.

Let us note here that there is nothing inherently more wonderful about the marathon as a race than there is about any other running event. Alas, the marathon has somehow become the glamour event in popular running, with the unfortunate result that far too many

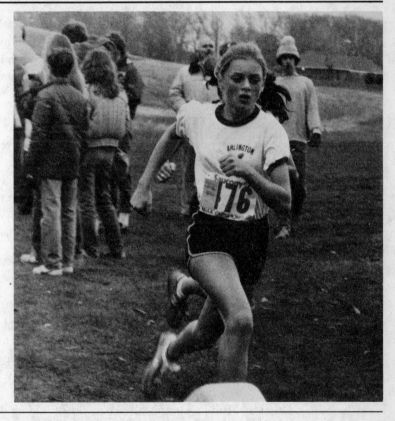

Talent often literally runs in a family: This is Coach Squires's niece, Karin. Your personal dedication to training and your determination to succeed play just as large a role in your running success as your genes, however. (Photograph from the authors' collection)

people run this race and overlook the joys of races to which they are better suited.

A muscle biopsy and full stress test might demonstrate your physical potential to excel at a given distance, but such tests in no way measure your psychological desire to excel.

ISOTONIC AND ISOMETRIC EXERCISES

These are basic types of exercises:

1. Isotonic exercises involve muscle contractions that produce movement through a partial or complete range of motion. In other words, they are concerned mostly with the development of muscle tone and strength, endurance, power, flexibility, balance, agility, and coordination. Examples include weight training and calisthenic exercises.
2. Isometric exercises also are for the purpose of developing muscle tone, size, strength, and power, but they involve no movement as such. Blood flow through the muscle tissues is constricted during an isometric exercise, so there's little effect on muscle or general endurance. Examples include tightening the fist, flexing the biceps muscle, pressing the palms together, and pushing against an immovable object such as a wall.

PROGRESSIVE RESISTANCE, PROGRESSION

Gains in strength through weight training are a result of these gradual increases in resistance. Resistance can be increased by adding weight, increasing the number of repetitions within sets or the number of sets, or by decreasing the rest time between sets.

Weight training traces its history back to Milo of Crotona, a Greek wrestler who trained by lifting a young calf across his shoulders daily and walking around a large stadium with it. As the calf turned into a bull, Milo grew stronger and the concept of progressive resistance was born.

There is a great deal of controversy over what kind of equipment is best. There are basically three options:

1. ***Free weights:*** This category includes dumbbells (short bars) and barbells (long bars) with adjustable cast-iron plates affixed to their ends. A good 110 lb. starter set, which is all anyone interested in tone and moderate strength gain needs, costs about $30 in a sporting goods store. Each set has individual plates weighing from 2.5 lbs. to 10 or 20 lbs.

2. ***Universal gym:*** This is a jungle-gym-like apparatus of weights and pulleys, with stations for leg, chest, and shoulder presses, latissimus pulls, curling, chinning, dipping, and hip flexions. You can learn to use a Universal in about twenty minutes. Most good gyms have them.

3. ***Nautilus machines:*** These are the latest in weight-training equipment. They were first used for rehabilitative work and by sports teams. Nautilus's major clients are still clinics and football teams, but more than 600 health clubs in the United States now have them.

   Each station consists of a giant metal and naugahyde frame into which the person using it is securely strapped. Each station works a single muscle group. What distinguishes Nautilus machines is that they work on a "cam" system of rotary motion. Each machine has a cam—a metal circle with an off-center hole—that varies the strength of the resistance according to the strength of the muscle as it goes through the motion of the machine. The cam is shaped like a chambered nautilus shell; hence the name. It gives the muscle a total workout throughout its entire range of motion.

Extravagant claims are made for the various types of weight training, but each person should experiment to find what suits him or her best. In general, free weights are recommended by serious trainers and athletes because free weights allow you to choose the desired range of motion. With Universal and Nautilus machines, you are locked into the movement path of the machine. On the other hand, free weights take technique. You must know how to balance and lift a weight in order not to injure yourself. Heavy free weights can be dangerous for the novice.

Most injuries in weight lifting are caused by "cheating," that is, by using jerking or explosive movements instead of just a steady lift. With Nautilus machines, you can't cheat. You're strapped in, and you have to do what the machine does.

The machines are best for rehabilitating injuries, for older people, and for normal people who are just interested in getting in shape, but for athletes they don't take the place of free weights. Free weights are the most specific and the fastest way to build strength. They give you a workout.

CIRCUIT TRAINING

This method combines aerobic exercises and weight training in a series of exercises done without rest. Choose ten to fifteen exercises and plan stations for them around the room. Each exercise should concentrate on a different part of the body. The whole plan is called a circuit, and the series should be performed without pausing. A variation of this plan is to do three or four shorter circuits consisting of different exercises with rest breaks between circuits. This plan makes weight training aerobic.

WEIGHT TRAINING

The physiological truth of the matter is that an increase in the size of your muscles in no way impairs the functioning of your joints. In fact, proper strength training involving slow, full-range movements actually increases flexibility. The only possible damage weight training can do to flexibility involves not the muscles, but the joints. Doing the exercises in an excessively fast or jerky fashion will cause joint damage. Furthermore, this approach will not increase strength or quickness (though some seem to think that it will). It is more important, therefore, to do all exercises with weights in a slow, smooth manner.

Proper strength training will develop and strengthen the muscles and tendons around the joints, thereby reducing the risk of stress-related injuries.

Running does not develop all of the leg muscles to the same degree. The hamstrings become highly developed, while the thighs and calves get relatively little development. Running also gives the upper torso muscles very little development, if any. The muscular imbalances caused by running often lead to injuries. Proper strength training can help to prevent such injuries by correcting imbalances.

In the event that you are injured and can't run, weight training can help to keep you in shape. Contrary to popular belief, weight training has significant cardiovascular benefits. These benefits are limited, of course, by the fact that less time can be spent on weight training than on running. Weight lifting normally should be done no more than three times a week for sessions lasting twenty minutes. Strength training may not keep a serious runner in shape, but it is much better shape than doing nothing. And for a person whose mileage is limited by chronic injuries, weight training may have the same cardiovascular effect as additional miles per week of running without the same risk of injury!

Many runners suffer poor form during the late stages of a run. The result may be a loss of efficiency, which hastens the onset of exhaustion. Strength training can help the distance runner's form in the final miles by providing a selective strengthening of the arms.

Proper weight training, which includes stretching, will not result in a loss of flexibility, or being muscle-bound. Right after a strenuous workout, a muscle may be engorged with blood, slightly swollen and less flexible, but this is a very temporary condition. Men can build muscle bulk; average women can't. Men have a much higher level of testosterone in their bloodstreams than women do, and testosterone is necessary to cause hypertrophy, or muscle growth. The potential for muscle in women is just one-tenth that of men.

There are two basic approaches to weight training: exercise machines and free weights (among which we would include not only the standard barbells and dumbbells, but also the weighted gloves now available for runners to wear during their roadwork). Both approaches to weight training offer their benefits and their drawbacks.

To understand the pluses and minuses of the different forms of weight training, it is first necessary to know which muscle groups the weight-training runner should be attempting to develop. These groups are the biceps, triceps, pectorals, trapezius, deltoids, latissimus dorsi, rectus abdominus, and transversus. It would be easier to say that you want to develop every muscle in your body that running does not, but you must learn to think of your body as not just "upper body" and "lower body," but in terms of the different muscle groups so that you will see how the various weight exercises act on the specific muscle group you want to develop. There is no one exercise that develops the entire upper body. Running develops the entire lower body, albeit unevenly.

Both exercise machines and free weights can develop any of the requisite muscle groups, but the two different approaches develop the muscles in slightly different ways. It is impossible for the athlete to injure himself or herself while exercising on a properly designed weight-training machine because the machine will not allow him or her to assume a posture or make a movement that could lead to injury. In short, the athlete is strapped into the machine and can only make certain movements. The problem is that the movements allowed by the machine may not exactly duplicate the movements the athlete makes while running (or practicing any other sport). Working out with the machine develops the desired muscle groups, but may not develop them in a way that is exactly transferrable to running.

The reverse of this is true with free-weight exercise. Unlike the machine, it is easy for free weights to injure the novice exerciser, but it is also very easy to duplicate the exact type and range of motion demanded by the sport while working out with free weights.

The smartest approach for the weight-training runner who has never before worked with weights is first to build him- or herself up using exercise machines, then phase in free-weight work. The fitter you are, the less likely you are to be injured. Join a club that offers machinery and ask the counselors there which machines will develop the muscle groups you want to build up. After several weeks of such a program, ask for guidance for proper free-weight technique. The best free-weight exercises for the muscle groups identified above are the bench press, the military press, the stiff-legged dead lift, bent-over rows, upright rows, barbell curls, and lying triceps extensions.

There are two other approaches to weight training that a novice can begin immediately and safely. One is the use of weighted gloves while running. The gloves, available in stores and also through the mail, have 8-ounce lead weights sewn into them, and have pockets to accommodate another 8-ounce weight. In other words, you can make the gloves weigh one pound or one-half pound. Even at a full pound, they don't feel very heavy when you put them on, but just try running a few miles in them. The nice things about the weight gloves are their simplicity, their duplication of the exact movements of running arm-use, and their light weight (which renders injury essentially impossible). You will have to experiment to determine just how far you can run with them, though. What are you going to do with two one-pound weights if you hit the halfway point in your workout and find you can no longer move your arms? Start out with the gloves at their lightest, and your workout mileage at its shortest, and work up gradually. The gloves are most effective when a person runs hard hill repeats, but only the truly fit athlete should try that. If you run without the gloves the day after such a workout, you'll feel like you could whiz right past Grete Waitz. (You probably in fact will not be able to, but you'll feel like it.)

The other approach to weight training is to use your body: do push-ups and sit-ups. You can do these exercises anywhere, anytime, thereby overcoming the main excuses for shirking. Perform only bent-knee sit-ups, so you strengthen your abdominal muscles. By doing straight-legged sit-ups, you may be calling on your thigh muscles. To enhance the training effect, do sit-ups on an inclined board, sitting up against gravity. To reduce the chance of getting a side-stitch, and, incidentally, to get rid of the flab on the sides of your waist, lie on your side and sit up sideways, touching your elbow (remember, put your hands behind your head for bent-knee sit-ups) to your buttocks. These side-raisers are tough. Try to do five of them on each side, then work up gradually.

Regarding push-ups, keep your back straight, lower your chest to the ground, and have your hands no farther apart than the width of your shoulders. (The closer together your hands, the harder it is to do the push-ups; the farther apart they are, the easier.) We recommend doing several sets of push-ups rather than doing too many of them. The reason is that your goal is not to build up bar-bending sheer strength, but instead to build up muscles that will allow you to move fast and keep moving fast. The rule of thumb for all weight training is: low weight and high number of repetition equals speed; high weight and low repetition equals brute strength. (Of course, the terms "low" and "high" weight are relative. What is high weight for you today may prove medium or low weight in a few years.) Trying to do high weight with high repetitions is like trying to run fast, long distance—impossible. You're only burning yourself out if you embrace such a program, and any experienced athlete who sees you will snicker. Avoid such mortification, not to mention discomfort.

Something else to avoid is doing any weight training before going out to run. Save such workouts for after the run, or for days off from running. Weight training builds up a great deal of lactic acid, the substance that makes your muscles feel tired. The last thing you need before even taking a step is to be awash in lactic acid. You might want to intersperse your warm-down stretching routine with sit-ups and push-ups; but don't run over to the local spa for a weight session and then try to race back home.

A CAUTIONARY NOTE ABOUT STEROIDS

Don't take them. You will do yourself a lot of harm, and probably no good.

Steroids are synthetic forms of testosterone, the male hormone. Testosterone gives men a muscle-building advantage over women. Too much of a good thing can be bad, however, and male athletes who have taken steroids run the risk of being thrown out of international competition for their use. Further, there is little scientific evidence (but a great deal of anecdotal—word-of-mouth—evidence, most of which can be chalked up to wishful thinking) that steroids increase strength in a man.

A woman athlete may be tempted to take steroids because they would seem to offer an equalizing factor between herself and male competitors. The scientific jury is still out on the question of whether or not steroids help a woman increase her strength. There is absolutely no scientific doubt that steroids impart a number of culturally undesirable male secondary sexual characteristics to women: Steroids make a woman's face and chest hair grow conspicuously. They deepen her voice. They cause acne. Steroids also may interfere seriously with a woman's sexual characteristics.

As Patricia Connolly, the outstanding former women's track coach at UCLA, put it, "The use of steroids does—I hate to say this, but it's true—make freaks out of women. Women are beautiful creatures the way God made them, and they can do a lot of things tremendously well. We don't even have any idea of how well we can do some things because we haven't been trying very long; but by taking male hormones, a woman is really changing what she is all about." The athlete who has confidence in his or her training, and the person who has confidence in himself or herself, will not take steroids.

MONONUCLEOSIS

The vast majority of people who get mononucleosis (mono) are between seventeen and thirty. Many people from lower socioeconomic groups are exposed to the virus as children and develop an immunity to it; those who haven't are most susceptible to the virus once they have moved into a communal setting. Even though mononucleosis is communicable, it is usually spread in airborne droplets from coughing and sneezing or through oral contact; it is not as infectious as flu and the common cold. It is contagious from just before the symptoms' appearance until the fever and sore throat are gone.

Mononucleosis is an infection of the lymph system and causes painful swollen glands in the neck, armpits, and groin; it can also affect the nervous system and the lungs. It varies in degree of severity; some people who have mononucleosis may think that they have the flu or a cold or that they're just feeling run-down. These cases can be cured by treating the symptoms like those of a cold or the flu.

It's important to stop physical activity and get plenty of rest in the early stages of mono because the spleen often becomes enlarged and can rupture if you overexert yourself. Hepatitis or severe sore throat and other secondary infections that require antibiotics can also develop.

TREATMENT OF COLDS

Studies have shown that a person who exercises regularly is as subject to colds and other infectious diseases as the person who doesn't. Most viruses are transmitted through the hands to the mucous membranes of the eyes and nose. If your hands come in contact with a surface that contains live cold viruses (doors, handrails, typewriters, books, another person's hand) and you then rub your eyes or put your fingers in your nose, you're likely to transmit the virus to mucosal areas where it will thrive. (Interestingly, colds are not usually transmitted by kissing, because the mucosa in the mouth and throat does not readily support viruses.)

If you catch a cold, vigorous exercise won't work it out. On the contrary, when you have a cold, strenuous exercise places an additional burden on the body when all its resources are needed to combat infection. The best thing to do is to take it easy when you have a cold.

What should you do for a cold or flu? The old remedy of rest, warmth, fluids, and aspirin is still your best bet. Be sure to drink lots of fluids, hot or cold.

The decision to stay home should be based on the severity of your symptoms. If you have a temperature higher than 100°F, if you have any severe symptoms, such as a bad cough or muscle aches, or if you feel you can't work, stay home.

Pamper yourself when you have a cold. Don't try to be a hero or heroine by going to work and sharing your bacteria with other people. The average person will fight off a cold in three or four days by taking it easy at home, getting plenty of rest, drinking more liquids than usual, and taking some aspirin, except in the case of a really bizarre type of infection. The person who attempts to continue business as usual may convert a common cold into an uncommon cold and may suffer not just a few days but weeks.

Aspirin, one of the greatest drugs ever discovered, takes away some of the aches and chills, reduces temperature, and helps the immune mechanisms. Exactly how and why aspirin works is a mystery, but it does work.

Liquid consumption should be increased to replace fluids lost through sweating, which is your body's way of getting rid of fever.

To protect yourself against colds and other viral infections, get the rest you normally need, eat a balanced diet, and get some exercise. A reasonably healthy body is better able to resist infections than a body that isn't so healthy. Avoid crowded places, where there is increased likelihood that you'll encounter some germ-carrying hero who should be home in bed. Dress sensibly when you go out in the cold and remember what your mother always told you: "Wear something on your head."

It's impossible to overemphasize the importance of dressing warmly. When your body gets chilled, your immune mechanism doesn't work the way it's supposed to work and germs that normally would be repulsed are able to get into your body and do their dirty work. Nowhere does this happen more often than in your nose, and for this reason it's important that you keep your head warm. Without a hat, you lose enormous amounts of body heat, and your nose is one of the first things to get chilled. When your nose gets cold, the lining stops secreting the mucous blanket that contains the bacteria-dissolving enzymes and your respiratory system loses its first line of defense.

When any one area of the body is chilled, the heart frantically pumps blood into that area in an attempt to warm it up. If you don't wear overshoes and if your feet get cold enough, the blood vessels will become so constricted in an attempt to hold in heat that it's impossible for sufficient blood to get to your feet. The result is frostbite.

Even if you don't get frostbite, your entire body temperature will be affected if any one part of your body is sufficiently chilled. It is at this point that resistance breaks down. The body is a finely tuned mechanism, and it doesn't take too much chill to put it out of tune and leave us most susceptible to colds.

Even dressing warmly may not be enough if you must be outside for long periods in brutally cold weather. What may be required is a change in diet to include more fats than you normally would consume. Fats give your body the extra calories it needs to keep your body temperature stabilized.

You don't have to worry too much about gaining weight from eating fatty foods because your body will burn up these extra calories to keep you warm. But don't forget to return to your sensible eating habits as soon as appropriate. Otherwise, you'll emerge in the spring looking like a butterball.

LOWERING BLOOD PRESSURE AND REDUCING INSOMNIA

Vigorous exercise is a good prescription for reducing high blood pressure, says a physician who knows about it firsthand.

Dr. J. Robert Cade of the University of Florida College of Medicine reports that he and associates were able to control 90 percent of high-blood-pressure cases through exercise alone or with smaller doses of drugs after a month of exercise.

The exercise involved either running twenty minutes, swimming twenty laps, or bicycling for about an hour three to five nights a week. Regular running brought Dr. Cade's blood pressure down from 150/105, which is rather high, to 100/60, which is very good.

Enough exercise to feel pleasantly tired is one of the best ways to conquer insomnia, but not right before bedtime. Tests at St. Louis University indicate that relaxation at that time is a better way to insure getting to sleep. But a good fast walk during the late afternoon or evening is fine. So is a jog, provided you are in shape.

SPORTS MEDICINE REPORT

The vast majority (60 percent) of injuries among long-distance runners (fifty miles per week or more) are the result of improper training. In one study, knee pain was the most common single complaint

(29 percent), followed by shin splints and Achilles tendonitis. Treatments recommended varied from rest or reduced mileage to routine stretching with attention to the hamstring and calf muscles and to properly fitting shoes with good shock-absorbing capacity.

Foot orthoses were prescribed in 46 percent of the cases; the results were beneficial in 78 percent of these cases. Pronation of the foot was found to be the way in which many runners compensate for their ailments. However, foot pronation serves only to provide short-term relief in most cases and often results in additional problems because of altered gait. Orthoses were found to be quite effective, particularly in relieving the secondary effects of compensatory foot pronation and those conditions associated with it, especially during the acute phase of the condition.

An orthosis is a supportive device fabricated from plastic, molded to the foot, and inserted in the shoe. The orthosis keeps the foot in a position where it will function most efficiently and with the least amount of stress on the joint, ligaments, and tendons. In many cases, it relieves irritation to the specific body part to allow for continued participation in sports during the healing process. An orthosis is made only on the order of the physician. The average orthosis lasts approximately six months to one year with normal use.

Another concern is Morton's foot (a condition in which the second toe is longer than the big one) or a high-arch foot. Telltale signs include a callus under the second or third metatarsal, a heel bump on the outside upper edge, the big toe pointing toward the little toe, and flat feet. If any of these are present, you have Morton's foot.

Since Morton's syndrome is permanent, a permanent treatment is usually indicated. Doctors who treat feet now have mechanical treatment methods that are comfortable and specific. The most permanent and efficient treatment for Morton's foot is a supportive (orthotic) device that is made over a cast of the foot and is thicker under the ball of the foot behind the first toe.

It is difficult to consider Morton's foot an abnormality because it occurs frequently; it is estimated that one-third of the general population has Morton's syndrome. It is just not an optimum condition for overdoing the sport of running.

5

GETTING STRONGER

The previous chapter provided basic information about strength and health for any runner. This chapter offers more advanced and specific advice for two different sorts of runners—the competitive racer and the person who runs for health and fitness.

How are these two types of runners different from one another in terms of their strength-training needs? Both the racer and the fitness runner will want to develop more upper-body strength than occurs as a result of running only, but the racer will want to spend most of the time he or she has available for training out on the roads actually running. Many fitness runners probably exercise in order to help themselves stay fit or remain at some model of physical appearance that they find attractive. This generally means they want uniform development between their upper and lower bodies. In turn, this means they will want to spend more time strengthening their arm and torso muscles than will the competitive racer.

Nevertheless, below are four strength-building techniques that both racer and fitness runner share. Before atempting any of these new exercises, you should be examined by a sports physician to make certain these additions to your training will not harm you. We urge such examination and approval for every one of the exercises described in this chapter. We also strongly advise you to find a competent exercise instructor who can demonstrate these techniques to you personally, and check your form.

Stationary Bicycles

Stationary bicycles are good tools to use to warm up before running or to maintain aerobic fitness when you can't run. They come in many forms, from the very inexpensive and unsophisticated to costly computerized marvels. Keep this range of choice in mind when selecting the type of stationary bike you need for the kind of workout you want.

An athlete just starting an exercise program rarely needs a sophisticated stationary bike. Generally, the more costly and sophisticated the bike, the greater the level of resistance it can be programmed to offer. A person who hits the anaerobic zone when jogging 15-minute miles does not need a stationary bike that can be programmed for high resistance. While such things as electronic timers, pulse readers, and the ability to simulate riding up and down hills can be pleasant diversions for any rider (more about diversions below), they are not absolutely necessary to athletic training. Getting your pulse into the aerobic zone *is*.

This is why the advanced runner is wasting his or her time by pedaling a stationary bike that cannot offer adequate resistance. One of us once burned up (yes! up in smoke!) two hard rubber resistance wheels on a rudimentary stationary bike before this obvious fact dawned on him. If it takes much more than 3 or 4 minutes of pedaling at the bike's maximum resistance level to get your pulse into your aerobic zone, it's the wrong bike for you. (Of course, this *does not* mean you should always set any bike at the max for any workout. If you can reach your aerobic level at a lower setting on a given machine, terrific.)

The automatic timers on these things don't always work well, so wear your stopwatch when riding a stationary bike. Also check the bike over carefully to see if there are any screws, bolts or other protrusions that might catch and cut you if you assume any position other than the normal seated riding one. One of us had the unique experience of gashing his knee open about 4 inches when, becoming a bit cramped in the hamstrings during a 2-hour bike workout, he stood up in the pedals as he did when riding a bike fast as a youngster, and found there was a long screw sticking out where it should not have been.

Finally, we must admit that riding a stationary bicycle—although outstanding supplementary and alternative exercise for any runner—rates a bit below watching grass grow on the list of stimulating human experiences. Riding a real bike is fun. Not so with one stuck in one place. We have found cable television the perfect solution to this problem, particularly the music-video channels. If this solution can't be applied in your situation, we suggest wearing a personal stereo. Having to ride a stationary bicycle with no visual and/or aural entertainment is about 100 times more mentally grueling than running the Western States 100-miler. Be nice to yourself.

Dips

Dips are a form of weight training that, like sit-ups and push-ups, use the athlete's own body weight to supply the resistance. It is, therefore, deeply satisfying to feel yourself being able to do a greater number of them as you become stronger—you can move *you* that many more times! Dips demand greater strength and coordination than do push-ups and sit-ups, and that's why we include them in this chapter.

You perform dips on parallel bars or a similar apparatus. Many gyms have a special station for dips. To perform the basic dip, place both hands in front of you, one on each of the parallel bars. You then push yourself up into the air until your arms are fully extended. Next, slowly lower yourself until your chest is level with the parallel bars. Then slowly push yourself back up again. Each time you *lower and raise* yourself, that's one dip. Perform as many dips as you can until you can no longer fully extend your arms. Then stop.

Dips strengthen many upper body muscles: the deltoids, shoulder muscles, upper pectorals, triceps, biceps, and laterals. They are one of the best all-around conditioners for any runner.

The advanced dip is performed exactly like the basic dip, except that now you place your hands behind you. This instruction does not mean that you turn your palms outward and grasp the bar behind your back. Your palms are still facing inward; you just move your hands backward from the basic dip position and grasp the bar behind your back instead of in front of your chest. As you'll discover,

DIPS

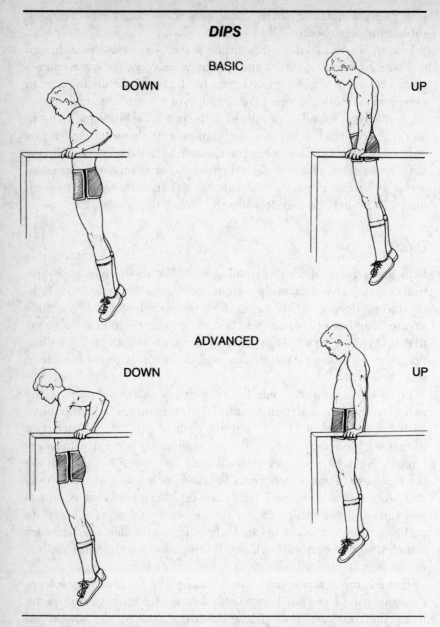

Although the dips shown here are performed on parallel bars, you may have other apparatus available that would be perfectly adequate for the exercise. Build up your strength with the basic dips before moving on to the advanced form.

advanced dips are lots harder to do than the basic variety. They are probably unnecessary for the competitive long-distance runner, although sprinters would benefit from them. The fitness runner who wants to explore the limits of upper-body weight training also benefits from advanced dips.

Shoulder Press

Both racers and fitness runners benefit from doing shoulder presses, because athletes in both categories will want to strengthen their deltoids. Shoulder presses isolate the shoulder muscle group: consequently, they're highly effective for its development.

The shoulder press can be performed with a barbell or on one of several different exercise machines designed for the purpose. (When performing it with a barbell, have another athlete "spot" you to prevent dropping the weight or otherwise injuring yourself.) You perform the press the same way with either kind of resistance mechanism: Lower the weight behind your neck to the top of your shoulders. Slowly push the weight upward until your arms are at full extension. Then slowly lower it to your shoulders again. When lifting a barbell, the bar must always remain parallel to your shoulders; you must avoid lifting up one end and then the other. Perform both lifting and lowering the bar slowly and smoothly. The slower you lift weights, the more benefit you gain from the exercise. Each time you lift and lower the weight counts as one repetition.

Abdominal Curls

It's extremely important for runners to strengthen their stomach muscles. Running greatly strengthens the back muscles, but does nothing for the gut. The stomach and back muscles balance each other in the torso, just as the quadricep muscles and hamstrings do in the legs. Imbalance between counterpoised muscle groups is one of the main reasons for injury in athletics. Your stomach muscles have to be as strong as your back muscles to prevent such an imbalance.

Sit-ups strengthen your stomach muscles, but abdominal curls strengthen them more. "Ab" curls also give significantly more definition to the stomach muscles, an ancillary benefit many athletes find aesthetically pleasing. Because ab curls are much more strenuous than sit-ups, please do not attempt them until you've been doing sit-ups regularly for a year or more. (The correct sit-up procedure is described in Chapter 4.)

To perform the ab curl, assume the same position that you use for a bent-knee sit-jup. To execute the ab curl, start to sit up very slowly, keeping your neck perpendicular to your torso. When you are from one-third to one-half sitting up (that is, your back forms an angle between 30 and 45 degrees with the floor), *stop*, and slowly and gently bend your head forward. You will feel your stomach muscles tighten up. Then straighten your neck so it is again perpendicular to your torso, and lie back down slowly. Hold the "up" position for 1 full second before going back down.

It's not necessary to scrunch your chin down into your chest when executing the "top" posture of the ab curl. Just bend your head forward until you feel your gut tighten.

Neither expect nor try to do as many ab curls as you can bent-knee sit-ups. Ab curls work the surface of the gut muscles much harder than sit-ups. They are, therefore, an excellent means of ensuring balance between stomach and back muscles when the back muscles have been strengthened by running hills.

Fitness runners may want to explore the benefits offered by advanced ab curls. (This advanced exercise is neither necessary nor recommended for the competition racer. Spend your time on the roads, instead.) To do the advanced version, assume the basic position, then lift your legs up until they're perpendicular to the floor. Point your toes right up to the ceiling. (You may find it easier to balance yourself if you cross one leg over the other at the ankles.) Then execute the ab curl as you would normally. Keep your legs straight up until you're done with your set.

This posture results in more rigorous exercise because holding your legs up completely eliminates your ability to use your hip flexor muscles even incidentally in performing the curl. All of the effort comes from the gut muscles—so take it easy if you decide to try ab curls this way.

Other Similarities between Weight Work for Racers and Fitness Runners

Two basic points about weight training apply to both racers and fitness runners. First, don't do exercises for your legs unless you've been advised by a sports medicine expert to do them. Even then,

ABDOMINAL CURL

BASIC

DOWN   UP

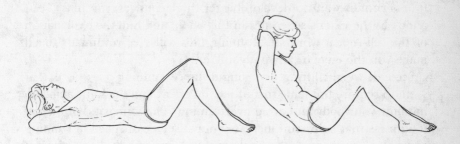

ADVANCED

DOWN   UP

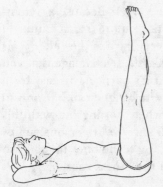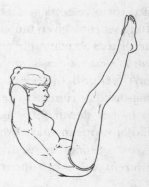

The obvious difference between the basic and advanced "ab" curl is that you do the latter with your feet straight up in the air. What's less apparent is how much harder the advanced ab curl is to perform. In both forms of ab curl, you should tuck your chin down toward your chest when you've stopped raising your upper body off the floor. You needn't scrunch your chin against your collarbone. A simple chin-tuck is sufficient and helps prevent a sore neck the next day.

don't do them unless that expert also knows what kind of running schedule you've been performing. Weight lifting leaves microscopic tears in your muscles. These tears leave your legs feeling stiff and sore when you run. Some other exercise physiologists disagree with us about this, but we've never seen them run seriously. Even fitness running gives your leg muscles all the work they need. If you as a fitness runner want to develop bigger thigh muscles, run hills. Take a look at the racer's schedules in this book, and find the explanation of the hill-repeat workout. Running hills will give you quads that'll make you the envy of any bodybuilder.

Second, weight lifting and long-distance running are sports that seem to require the same sort of mental effort and the same ability to monitor your body and avoid overtraining. The same kind of mental toughness that helps you increase your distance or speed in running also helps you through the final repetition in a weight-lifting set. But we want to caution you to remember an extremely important difference between these two sports: Weight lifting is always anaerobic, while long-distance running is rarely anaerobic. The term "anaerobic" means that your muscles are receiving oxygen inadequate for the work they are performing. As a runner, you've probably come to think of "anaerobic" as meaning a period when you've been breathing hard for a reasonable amount of time, or longer. Because a weight-lifting set for a given muscle group rarely takes more than a minute to complete, you may well not be breathing very hard at the end. *But the muscles you've exercised are still minutely damaged.* It's damage that you don't feel until the next day. We find that it's particularly easy for a long-distance runner to get carried away with weight training, only to his or her detriment. Take it very easy when starting out with this kind of supplementary exercise and get to know your personal limits.

Now let's look at specific strength-building techniques for the two different classes of runner, the racer and the fitness runner.

STRENGTH FOR THE RACER

Cross-Country Skiing Machines

This machine is one of the big secrets of serious racers. It duplicates the benefits of cross-country skiing, just as the stationary bicycle duplicates the benefits of bicycling. Unlike bicycling, cross-country skiing works the entire body. The exercise not only offers even greater aerobic benefits than running, it develops the athlete's muscles that help him or her as a runner—and it does this without the pounding of running. This machine is ideal for an injured racer to maintain fitness. It is superior to actual cross-country skiing for such rehabilitative purposes because the athlete remains indoors, unexposed to the stressful climate often associated with cross-country skiing.

Running in a Swimming Pool

This is a technique used by elite racers to maintain or even improve their strength and fitness when injured. Wearing or holding a flotation device, the runner goes into the deep end of a full swimming pool and "runs" while floating in place. Because water is 800 times denser than air, it requires considerable effort to attain anywhere near one's normal leg speed in this workout. The exercise can therefore result in increased aerobic capacity, while offering the advantage of exercising exactly those muscles used in running. The exercise is normally used only by injured runners because, although it avoids any pounding or muscular strain, it is both boring and not easy to set up.

Weighted Gloves

We described these gloves and their basic use in Chapter 4. We mention them again here because they're an outstanding strength-building tool for the serious racer. These gloves confer their greatest benefits to the racer when worn for hill repeats, intervals, and the weekly long run. Their benefits are as much psychological as physiological—you feel so much *lighter* without them! We don't recommend wearing the weighted gloves all the time. Twice a week would be plenty; thrice weekly, the maximum.

Other Supplementary Exercises

We don't recommend that the racer perform any other supplementary exercises, unless so advised by his or her coach, trainer, or sports physician.

In Chapter 4, we mentioned free-weight exercises in addition to those we have already discussed in depth in this chapter. They were the bench press, stiff-legged dead lift, bent-over rows, upright rows, barbell curls, and lying triceps extensions. These are indeed excellent conditioning exercises for runners in general, but we have not found them to be valuable for competitive long-distance racing. The dip, described earlier in the chapter in both basic and advanced forms, exercises all the muscle groups isolated by the free-weight exercises we're urging you to ignore. The dip also develops the latissimus dorsi, important muscles for proper arm carriage.

Sprinters *can* benefit from these free-weight exercises, but long-distance racers are better advised to spend the time they would devote to performing them doing roadwork and resting instead. Sprinters may want to read the following section, where further exercise for these specific muscle groups is discussed.

STRENGTH FOR THE FITNESS RUNNER

Arm Curls

You can perform arm curls with either a barbell or dumbbells. There are also various exercise machines designed for arm curls. Free weights allow you to perform curls through a greater range of motion, beginning with your arms nearly straight down in front of you (if using a barbell) or your hands at your sides, well below your hips (if using dumbbells).

Because of the difference in range of motion available between free-weight curls and those done using a machine (where you begin with your arms bent at the elbow), you'll probably be able to lift more weight when doing curls on a machine. We suggest that you employ both methods of doing arm curls, if they're available to you. In weight lifting, range of motion is just as important to developing strength as is the weight of the resistance. We think dumbbells are superior to barbells in performing arm curls as a free-weight exercise. First, dumbbells allow for a greater range of motion. Second, dumbbells work each arm independently, so each arm lifts exactly the same weight. An experienced weight lifter using a barbell would know if he or she were "cheating" by using a strong arm to compensate for a weaker one, but the novice probably would not be so sensitive. If curling with dumbbells, always use the same amount of weight for each arm, even if one arm is stronger than the other (which is common). The weaker arm will catch up with the stronger arm, eliminating the imbalance. Whether using dumbbells or a barbell, keep your elbows pressed against your sides for maximum benefits.

Bench Press

Like arm curls, the bench press can be performed with either a barbell or with several different machines. We urge you to use the machine version of the exercise. Some machines offer almost exactly the same range of motion as using a barbell would provide. Some machines also duplicate performing the bench press with dumbbells, ensuring that you make the same effort with both arms. All machines provide the safety factor of preventing the weight from crashing down on you if you lose control.

You perform the bench press by lying on your back, usually on a bench, appropriately enough, and lifting a weight from your chest straight up into the air until your arms reach full extension. Even when using a machine, this technique demands some expertise. Make certain you position the bench so your chest is directly beneath the bar. Flex your knees and place your feet on the bench, in the bent-knee sit-up posture—or, better, raise your feet slightly off the bench. *Do not* leave your feet flat on the floor, or you'll unconsciously use your legs to help your pectorals push the weight up. (Lifting your feet into the air eliminates this problem altogether, but some people feel they look silly doing it. On the other hand, they have great pectoral muscles.)

There are also a variety of exercise machines that exercise the pectorals. If you're a member of a gym or health club, ask your instructors to explain which of these are available to you.

The remaining strength-building exercises for the fitness runner are all performed on exercise machines. There are numerous free-weight exercises for working the same muscle groups, but to tell you how to do them safely and correctly would require more exposition than we can provide here. If you're interested, join a good gym with good instructors.

BENCH PRESS

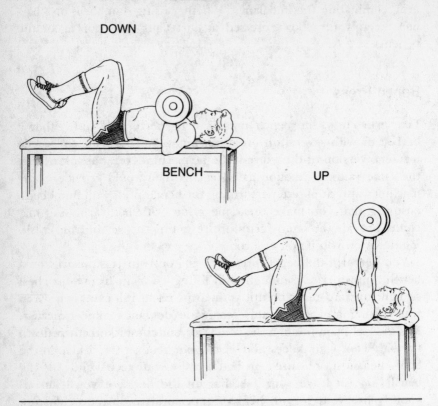

DOWN

BENCH—   UP

These drawings illustrate bench-press form with a free weight. Note that the feet are held slightly off the bench to prevent "cheating" with the leg muscles in lifting the barbell. If you use an exercise machine for doing bench presses, you may find that the weight is held higher in the air than it is here because machines vary in their design.

Lat Pull

The lat (shoulder blade) muscles not only help runners with their arm carriage, they give the body a look of power—or not, if the lats are puny. You already have several exercises to develop your lats (push-ups, dips, bench presses). Here's another—one that works them the hardest of all, while also helping develop the deltoids.

The lat pull machine is a bar hung through an overhead pulley by a rope. Weights are attached to the other end of the rope, providing the exercise's resistance. There are several different postures you can assume for doing this exercise, but the one we've found works the best is to sit directly beneath the center of the bar with your feet flat on the floor and your legs bent. It's the kind of position you'd reach in the "up" mode in a bent-knee sit-up, except that your hands are not clasped behind your head. They're reaching straight up over your head to grasp the bar.

Use your body weight to help you lower the bar to the point where you can assume the seated posture with your arms fully extended above you. When starting out with this exercise, pull the bar down in front of you until level with your chest. To perform the lat pull at an advanced level, pull the bar down behind your head until it is level with your shoulders.

Triceps Press

The apparatus for this exercise is basically the same as that for the lat pull. It is called a "press" because you push the weight down instead of pulling it down.

Stand facing the bar. Grasp it at either end and pull it down until level with the top of your chest. Now comes the important part: Tuck your elbows tight up against your sides and keep them there all through the workout. Then push the bar down as far as your arms will reach when tucked into your sides, raise it slowly back up to the top of your chest, and repeat 9 more times. (If you can do more than 10 repetitions of this or any other weight-lifting routine—except for those using your own body as the resistance—you should move on to a higher resistance level. Add more weight.)

By tucking your elbows against your sides, you isolate your triceps muscles and force them to move the weight. If you held your arms normally, you'd inadvertently bring in your shoulder, chest, and back muscles, defeating the purpose of the exercise.

Make sure you have good standing posture when performing the triceps press. Spread your feet apart to give you a firm base.

STRETCHING

Both the racer and the fitness runner who indulge in supplementary strength-building workouts should stretch the muscles in the upper body, just as they stretch their leg muscles, as part of their running.

The strength-building exercises we've suggested aren't likely to result in the overuse syndromes associated with the extreme repetitive motion of long-distance running, so stretching the muscles worked by them is not as much a form of preventive maintenance as it is in running. Nevertheless, stretching helps promote healing in muscles stressed by anaerobic exercise by promoting blood flow in them. It also feels good—which is reason enough to stretch.

Because stretching the upper body almost always involves the spine, it is *extremely important* that the athlete masters the proper posture for each stretch. Misaligning the spinal column introduces a whole lot of problems you don't want. Therefore, find an expert in stretching and work with him or her to develop a stretching routine that is appropriate for your strength-building exercises.

We will give you two simple, basic upper-body stretches. For your own sake, do them gently until you have a feel for proper posture.

1. *Hanging stretch:* Find a sturdy overhead object that you can grasp with both feet still on the floor. The top of a doorjamb often works well. So would a lowered chinning bar. Hold the bar (or whatever) firmly with both hands, then bend your knees so your legs support less and less of your weight. Do this slowly. Don't just jump at the bar and hang from it like an ape. Hold the posture for as long as feels comfortable, then straighten your legs to resume full support of your weight.

2. *Bent-over stretch:* Find a sturdy object about level with your waist, or even slightly higher. A dancer's stretching bar is ideal. Stand about 4 feet away from the bar, facing it. Lean forward and place both hands firmly on top of the object, or grasp it if possible. Your hands should not be close together. Place them the width of your shoulders apart, or a bit farther. Your neck should be perpendicular to your torso, meaning you're looking down at the floor. Hold this posture until it feels comfortable. (It probably won't, at first.) Then, keeping your neck perpendicular to your torso, lower your upper body farther down toward the floor. Do this very gently and slowly. Keep your legs straight all the while. When you feel your hamstring muscles tighten, stop, and hold the posture for as long as it feels comfortable.

6

MENTAL/EMOTIONAL ASPECTS OF RUNNING

It is widely known that running confers a multitude of mental and emotional benefits. What is not as widely understood is that a deep understanding of the athlete's intellectual and psychological mechanisms translates into vastly improved athletic performance. The interaction between psyche and body is a two-way street: The jogger works out at least partly to relieve depression and enhance self-esteem. The runner brings mental concentration and creative inspiration to his or her workouts in order to run with higher quality. The serious athlete must train the mind simultaneously with training the body, for races are won in the mind before the starting signal is given.

WHAT RUNNING DOES TO THE MIND

Science documents running's efficacy for reducing cases of minor depression and tension. Running will *not* be very helpful in cases of major emotional problems; indeed, taking into account the compulsive personality types running tends to attract, an increasing incidence of running programs *contributing* to depression, tension, and other emotional ailments can be expected. *Running is not a panacea for personal troubles.* If you have such problems, it is in your own best interests to consult a professional counselor. Personal observation suggests, however, that the great majority of running athletes accrue mental and emotional benefits from their sport. For the typical runner the most serious emotional strain connected with running comes from non-running friends asking him or her please to talk about something—anything—other than "jogging"!

Medical studies have shown that after twenty-five minutes of exercise the runner's brain "opens up," inspired by extra oxygen. The result is a very pleasant physical and emotional state. (Please don't look for the so-called "runner's high," though. Like many other types of peak experience, the "runner's high" is oversold to the novice. It is *not* a sudden alteration of consciousness resulting in a feeling of ecstatic dissociation from reality; on the contrary, the "high" that comes from running (1) builds gradually, (2) causes the athlete to *focus on*—not dissociate from—immediate reality, and (3) results from the runner's increased self-esteem in meeting goals he or she has established and in reveling in the integration of mind and body.) Some doctors now prescribe a daily jog to treat cases of minor depression. People who exercise feel better, look better, and perform better at their jobs. This may be the reason so many people are involved in running, even those who run for running's—not for competition's—sake.

The mental and emotional benefits derived from running are also generated by other sorts of aerobic exercise. What mechanism is involved in producing these benefits? The answer is unclear, but scientists believe that biochemical factors as well as purely psychological phenomena are at work. Exercise apparently triggers the production of the hormone epinephrine, a natural painkiller that is similar in chemical makeup to heroin and which, like the narcotic, gives pleasure while masking pain. Exercise may also work its magic by raising the body's temperature or by changing the cerebral blood flow, possibly in a manner that promotes the production of alpha waves by the brain (alpha waves are associated with relaxation and creative thinking).

Although any aerobic exercise will confer these benefits in certain amounts, running is one of the most effective ways to experience such pluses. Running is excellent training for the cardiovascular system because the exercise uses the largest muscles in the body, the leg muscles, and so it demands large quantities of blood and oxygen. This demand requires the heart to work harder than usual, and the heart, like any other muscle, becomes stronger, more efficient, and more resilient when training correctly and with respect.

Correct training also enhances one's *self-respect*. The runner initially derives personal satisfaction from setting and achieving difficult athletic goals (in terms both of performance and personal appearance and weight); but a runner eventually enjoys a more global sense of satisfaction when he or she realizes the strengths gained strictly through running are applicable to most other aspects of life. A hard day on the job doesn't seem quite as nerve-wracking when a person knows what it's like to sweat out hard mile after hard mile while practicing a mere hobby. An unexpected demand made by a friend becomes a totally minor inconvenience when compared to an unexpected, steep hill at the 25-mile mark in a marathon. The outbreak of a major war is most certainly less provoking than the outbreak of a major blister. Running helps the individual keep life's problems in perspective.

WHAT THE MIND DOES TO RUNNING

An interesting conversation once took place between Steve Scott, America's most outstanding miler of the late 1970s and early '80s, and Herb Elliott of Australia, arguably the greatest miler yet in history. Scottie asked Herb, "What do you think the ultimate time is for a mile?" and Elliott replied:

> There's probably going to be a quantum leap forward when we understand our minds better. I believe that we just barely understand our physical capabilities at this stage of the game. There will come a time when knowledge of ourselves will enable us to tap that physical resource. At that time, we'll see a quantum leap in all sports. . . . I see three minutes as a possibility, but not with our current knowledge.

Once a certain, relatively minimal level of physical fitness is reached, athletic performance derives largely from the athlete's mental/emotional attitude. Kenya's great Henry Rono, who set four world distance-running records in 1979, once said that when he finally met the man who could beat him in a race, he would not even have to watch the fellow run; he'd know the other man could beat him simply by speaking with him and sensing the intensity of his personality.

To be sure, the relatively minimal level of physical fitness necessary for peak athletic performance is, insofar as the non-gifted athlete is concerned, a relatively *high* level of fitness. The new distance runner must not put the psychic cart before the horse of hard scientific physical training; however, even the novice athlete can train his or her mind simultaneously with training his or her body. The purpose of an intense workout is, in fact, more to train the mind than it is to train the muscles and/or cardiovascular system. You can get all the aerobic benefits anyone could want by never exceeding 75 percent of your predicted maximum pulse rate—but you will *never* learn how to race by doing only such training. In short, if you haven't reached the minimal requisite level of physical conditioning, no amount of positive thinking is going to make you a racer; but there is no reason you cannot reach that physical level at the same time as you reach the requisite psychic level. Don't train your body at the expense of your mind.

Distance running is commonly associated with pain, but the champion runner knows this popular association is essentially balderdash. The serious racer will consider framing the following quotation from Henry Rono, who is certainly qualified to comment on the subject. Rono said: "If you train only to *take* the pain, you will never be any good; but if you train to *break* the pain, you can move on to a new level." Far too many runners seem willing to accept pain as a necessary component of competition and training. The runners who refuse to accept the pain, who fight back against it and bend it to their own wills, are champions.

In his excellent novel about a world-class miler, *The Olympian*, Brian Glanville writes about the miler's coach commenting on what the coach calls "the pain barrier." The coach observes:

> The athlete grows with each new conquest of pain, both as a runner and as a human being. He cannot *court* pain in a race, as he can in training, but if he is required to run through the pain barrier and he succeeds, then his performance will inevitably improve. . . . You cannot *see* it. . . . It is not like barbed wire. It does not resemble the water barrier in the steeplechase. . . . The pain barrier represents the physical limits beyond which an athlete thinks he cannot push himself, [but can], if he is prepared to accept the pain involved. . . . It is both physical *and* psychological."*

*Brian Glanville, *The Olympian* (Boston: Houghton Mifflin, 1980), p. 77.

Many runners, having read this far, are probably shaking their heads and muttering, "But the athletes this guy and Rono are talking about are gifted mentally as well as physically." You are right: They are. It is also correct that no individual has any control over Mother Nature's physical gifts; but it is just as correct that *every* individual exercises *enormous* control over his or her *own* psychological makeup. Consider, for example, the importance of the placebo effect in medical science. A placebo is, normally, a chemically inert substance (e.g., a pill made of milk-sugar). From a strictly physical perspective, it cannot possibly have any effect on a serious illness. Time and again, however, science has noted and admitted that, if a subject is given a substance by researchers and told how the substance will affect him or her (even if the researchers lie, which is often; never trust a researcher), the subject will often undergo exactly (or very nearly) the reactions he was told to expect. Further, many reactions to placebos are not merely imaginary—there are concrete, clinically verifiable changes accompanying them in the subject's body.

The operative mechanism in the placebo effect is the subject's *belief*. What the individual believes in such instances is not in him- or herself, but in the bogus powers of the sugar-pill. But one need not focus on a placebo in order to have faith—especially not to have faith in oneself. The patient who is cured by a placebo has actually been cured by the power of his or her own mind. The more clinical psychologists—especially those working in the field of parapsychology—gather empirical data on the workings of the mind, the more evidence there is that it is *imagination* that is both the single most powerful and most unique of all human powers. If an athlete *believes* he can break 40 minutes for 10,000 meters, he or she stands an excellent chance of actually running under 40 minutes for the distance. Even more certain, the athlete who does *not* believe he or she can break the 40-minute barrier will *never break it (on an accurate course)*.

What is the secret of achieving the proper emotional attitude for running success? There are probably two secrets. First, the athlete must be able to *visualize* achieving the desired goal. Picture yourself crossing the line beneath a huge digital clock reading the time you want to run on it. First, in other words, comes the *emotionally integrated* (not the *wishful*) belief that he or she *will inevitably succeed*.

Second comes the understanding that pain is a challenge, a mere

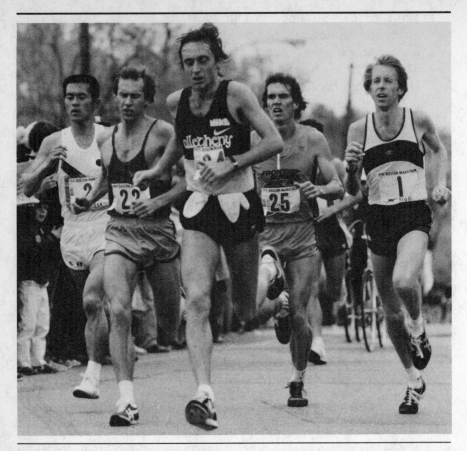

The leaders in the 1981 Boston Marathon show a range of facial expressions: Toshihiko Seko (#2), implacable concentration; Craig Virgin (#25), ferocity; Bill Rodgers (#1), optimism. (Photograph by Bill Boyle)

obstacle to a desired goal, and *not* a *barrier* to the goal. Studies contrasting the personalities of Formula One racing drivers with ordinary people suggest a way to achieve this goal, as do Rono's words. In the study of racing drivers and non-racing drivers, each subject was presented with a maze, the paths of which were lined with electrified metal strips. Each subject was also given an electrified stylus with which to attempt to trace a path through the maze. The goal was to trace the correct path through the maze in the shortest possible time; whenever the stylus touched one of the walls of the path, a time penalty was electronically added to the subject's total.

Each individual, racers and non-racers alike, was given two tries at the maze. The first attempt was made under ideal conditions: good lighting, a quiet environment, and a researcher standing by who kept encouraging the person. The second attempt was made under deplorable conditions: lights blinking unexpectedly on and off, horns and gongs going off at odd intervals, and a researcher who constantly berated the best efforts of the subject. Not surprisingly, most people performed far worse on the second attempt at the maze than they did the first time around, even though, with the learning experience of the initial maze run-through, they should have done better. Had conditions been ideal, they undoubtedly would have done better.

The Formula One drivers were the exception: Not only did their performance not deteriorate the second time through the maze, *it improved!* To repeat: the racing drivers' performance *improved* as the situation became *more stressful.* They rose to the challenge. They broke the barrier. How? *Most likely by focusing in on breaking the barrier as a personal reward.* We, as yet, have no idea what our mental limits are; remember what Herb Elliott said. Personal observation indicates that most people stay at a certain level of performance (in any field, not just running) because they think it's too much effort to rise to a higher level. Personal observation also has shown, time and again, how surprised those who *did* struggle to a higher level were that *it was so easy to do,* once the initial mental/emotional commitment was made. If you can train yourself to respond positively to the challenge of running uphill while your rivals die, there is no reason on earth why you cannot also learn to respond positively to the other great stresses (both physical and psychological) you'll encounter in racing. Most people respond negatively to stress. Most people are not champions.

One final point: The mind remains essentially trained, even when the body de-conditions due to injury or other impediments. The mind, however, will try to forget how to respond positively to pain, if given the chance. In practical terms, this means that if you haven't run truly hard for a long time, you'll probably flinch from doing a quality workout again—but you will remember how to confront stress successfully (and enjoy confronting it) the instant you begin your first hard pick-up. That is a fact. The body can get fat, but a trained athletic mind remains trained forever—which is why the athlete must be cautious about trying to come back from injuries too fast.

This fact also demonstrates why it is *stupid* to try to continue to run while seriously injured. Working out in constant pain only conditions the mind to *hate running,* and it also foolishly prolongs injury. Think of all the superstar runners who never seemed really to come back from a prolonged injury they also tried to "train through." Even though their bodies are now healed, their unconscious minds remember and resent all the pain associated with running.

Finally, the reason you should run only a few marathons annually has a deeper basis in psychology than in physiology. Your body recovers from the rigors of a marathon after only a few weeks, provided you had achieved the requisite level of initial fitness. Your mind takes about three months to recover from the stress.

The Greek ideal of the "whole person" was, of course, to have a sound mind in a sound body. Long-distance running can work wonders on the mind, but the mind can work literal miracles on long-distance running. Go for it!

7

PREVENTING INJURIES AND OTHER RUNNING PROBLEMS

COMMON RUNNING POSTURE PROBLEMS

Most of these problems can be seen in photographs taken while you are running. Make an effort to correct them.

1. *Overstriding:* Concentrate on a shorter and slightly faster arm swing. Consciously shorten the stride by shortening the forward reach of the foot.
2. *Incorrect knee lift:* Concentrate on lifting the knees just high enough for the feet to clear the ground during the recovery phase. Lifting knees any higher results in wasted energy. Long-distance running tends to bring the knees down where they belong. Be aware of knee lift constantly to be sure that you are not wasting energy through excessive lift. Correct this fault while doing pick-ups.
3. *Arms too high:* Study the correct arm movements and concentrate on these actions during running. Holding the palms of the hands inward and upward will help to keep the elbows close to the sides where they belong.
4. *Tightness in the hands, arms, and shoulders:* Work on quickstep drills during warm-up. Concentrate on keeping the hands,

arms, and shoulders loose during the drills. Keeping the fingers loose forces relaxation during long training runs.

5. *Bounce too high:* Lengthen the strike to the back by concentrating on leaving the foot in contact with the ground longer, after it passes under the center of gravity. Also, land lower on the ball of the foot. Stress a reaching action with the arms rather than a pumping action. Increase body lean slightly. Stress lower knee lift, and concentrate on keeping the head in the same plane while running.

6. *Landing on the heels:* Be conscious of the error and concentrate during practice sessions on the correct foot-ground contact. Shorten the stride slightly in order to avoid overreaching. Also, it might be beneficial to increase body lean slightly.

7. *Arm action:* The faster you swing your arms, as long as the action is rhythmic, the faster you will be able to move your legs. While sprinting, keep your arms low and pump them hard rapidly. For slower running, hold your arms in a comfortable, restful position, and keep their action to a minimum. Your hands should be fairly close to your chest, about at the height of the pectoral muscles. This posture minimizes the work the heart must do to pump blood and oxygen into the arms. Lower each hand and arm no more than a foot or so as the leg on the opposite side goes back. Out-of-rhythm flailing by either arm will also cause a similar, compensatory activity by the opposite side of the body. This motion is both tiring and inefficient. On the other hand, a runner whose legs have gone dead can often keep moving rapidly by pumping the arms as fast as possible.

8. *Breathing:* For anything less than a full sprint, breathing should be steady and rhythmic. You should inhale and exhale through a partially open mouth as well as through the nose. It is best to set up a breathing pattern. Anyone other than a trained athlete should probably breathe on a two-count beat. In other words, exhale every second time the right foot strikes the ground. If you are doing a lot of fast starting and stopping, remember to breathe very deeply when you get winded. A trick used by some of the distance runners at Oregon is to hold air in the cheeks for a brief instant before exhaling it with a brief "puff." The theory is that slightly pursing the lips

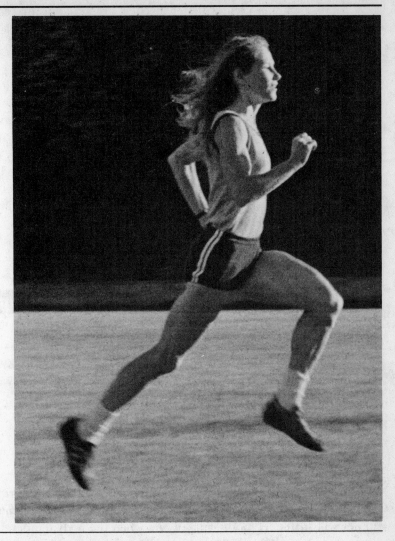

Running form: Doris Brown Heritage, the greatest woman long-distance runner in American history, demonstrates proper technique. Note the head held high, shoulders relaxed, fluid arm motion, loose fingers, and body weight landing evenly back toward the heel. (Photograph courtesy of Cal Fanders)

upon exhaling creates better alveolar pressure and makes for a longer and better oxygen-carbon dioxide exchange.

"THE STITCH"

"The stitch" is a temporarily severe pain located near the lower rib cage and adjacent abdominal area. Usually, the pain on the right side is particularly intense when the athlete inhales.

An athlete stricken with "the stitch" has two proven methods of relieving the condition. The first method is to bend forward at the waist as far as possible. This remedy can be used while continuing to run. The second solution is to stop running, lie on your back, and raise your arms above your head.

Possible reasons for "the stitch" are: eating too close to practice, overeating, intestinal gas or constipation, weak abdominal muscles, poor conditioning, and faulty breathing techniques during exertion. This last problem can be prevented by learning to tighten and relax the diaphragm while running. Slowing your pace is often quite helpful, too. Generally, "stitches" can be cured en route, without having to stop running. Undertraining for especially stressful running may also be a factor to consider, especially when we consider that very few accomplished athletes are bothered by "stitches."

HEAT CAN BE AN ENEMY

Hypothermia can strike any runner, in any kind of shape, during a race or hard workout—and *not only* the unconditioned, unacclimated runner will suffer. Hypothermia occurs when the body temperature falls below 95°F. The victim becomes increasingly apathetic and lethargic. Below 90°F coma can occur.

Hypothermia can occur when you don't expect it. A rapid decrease in body temperature occurs when the body's natural cooling mechanism—evaporation—stops because the body has lost too much fluid through sweating. Research has shown that the rate of loss of body fluids does not substantially change from temperatures of 70°F upward. A temperature of 60°F and high relative humidity can be just as dangerous as 90°F and low humidity.

What can be done to minimize the effects of heat on a runner?

1. During hot weather, keep body contents of magnesium and potassium high. These minerals occur naturally in foods such as bananas, watermelon, tomatoes, carrots, and cucumbers.
2. Wear cool clothes. Loose-fitting cotton, tank-top T-shirts with large breathing holes are best. Avoid nylon shirts because they retain heat. Wear a brimmed hat that shades your face.
3. Cool off *before* a race. You might as well start with a slightly depressed temperature.
4. Before a race, drink plenty of fluids. The American College of Sports Medicine suggests drinking twelve fluid ounces fifteen minutes before competition.
5. Drink plenty of fluids during a race and afterwards. Drink frequently during the race. Toss water on your body during a race to aid evaporation and cooling of the body.
6. Most important, schedule hard races for times when you'll be most likely to run well. Avoid races that start late in the morning or during the afternoon in the summer and hot-weather months of spring and fall.

Tips to Prevent Heat Injury

1. Try to schedule your workouts in the cooler hours of morning or evening. If possible, avoid the hours 10 A.M. to 2 A.M. and later races if the temperature and humidity are high.
2. Wear lightweight, loose-fitting clothing.
3. Do light warm-ups first, so that your body can gradually get used to the heat.
4. Drink liquids frequently (at least every hour). Commercially prepared fluids such as ERG are quite good.
5. Memorize the signs and symptoms of heat injury and be prepared to give proper first aid when necessary.
6. Hot weather and running don't mix unless you drink water before starting and continue with water along the way.
7. Drink a glass of water before running in temperatures of 80°F and higher.
8. If running more than six miles, provide for one or two stops along the way.

First Aid for Heat Problems

Heat stroke (dry skin) can be deadly

Symptoms:
1. Warm, dry skin
2. Abnormal breathing
3. Fast, weak pulse
4. Red-hot forehead

Treatment:
1. Move victim into the shade
2. Remove his/her clothes
3. Place victim on his/her back, head and shoulders elevated
4. Lower body temperature with ice bath or cold water
5. Fan the water to speed evaporation
6. Give the victim cool water
7. Get medical help quickly

Heat exhaustion (moist skin and thirst)

Symptoms:
1. Dizziness
2. Confusion
3. Fatigue
4. Excessive thirst
5. Cool, moist skin

Treatment:
1. Move victim to cool place
2. Remove his/her clothing
3. Give him/her a cool bath
4. Provide salty liquids
5. Rest 24 to 48 hours

Heat cramps

Symptoms:
1. Muscle spasms in abdomen, arms, legs
2. Severe cramping
3. Weak, nauseous

Treatment:
1. Move victim to cool area
2. Provide liquid ERG
3. Rest up to 48 hours

COLD PRESENTS PROBLEMS

Each of the seasons has special joys and each presents special problems to the runner. During the winter, runners contend with cold temperatures, poor road conditions, and an attitude that makes them want to stay indoors.

Although cold is the most obvious problem, it is the easiest to solve. Running generates tremendous amounts of body heat and, with appropriate clothing, you can stay warm even when it's near 0° F. The real difficulty is in the variability of temperature. Furthermore, body temperature may fluctuate widely, depending on the amount of sunlight, your direction with relation to the wind, humidity, and how much you are sweating.

A five-minute warm-up session of calisthenics before you put on your sweats and go out is important. Check temperature, wind speed, and direction before you start. Try to run initially into the wind and then run with the wind coming home. The reason for this rule is that even in the coldest temperatures almost everyone begins to sweat if he or she is adequately dressed. If you run away from the wind first, when you turn into the wind, you will have not only a twenty-to thirty-degree temperature drop to deal with, but also the cooling effect of sweat evaporating rapidly, a condition that can be uncomfortable and even dangerous. Furthermore, the end of a long run, when fatigue sets in, is not the time to be fighting a brisk winter wind and below-zero chill factors. Also be aware of the time of day. The shifts in temperature between 3:30 and 4:30 P.M. on a winter afternoon can magnify the problems of wind.

It is obvious that the usual clothes for cold weather are not appropriate for running not only because they are too bulky and make movement difficult, but also because they do not allow you to adjust to changes in body temperature or wind.

Multiple layers of thin clothing provide greater warmth and flexibility than a single heavy garment. The layer closest to the body should be soft and absorbent. For outer layers, woolens are ideal. A sweatshirt and pants over a T-shirt and shorts should suffice for 40° F days. A hat, turtleneck, and long johns or panty hose can be added at 30°F, a windbreaker at 10°–20°F, and extra socks, extra underpants, an extra T-shirt, and perhaps a face mask at 0°–10°F.

Hands, face, ears, and, in men, genitalia demand special protection against frostbite, which can affect these body parts when the rest of the body is warm. A headband worn underneath a hat to cover forehead and ears is valuable, for you can pull it down over your nose as a quickie face mask. Even in gloves, your fingers can become very cold. Warm ski gloves or wool mittens in which you can make a fist can be very helpful. A second pair of gloves or mittens (or even pulling a pair of socks over mittens) will make a noticeable difference.

It is important to be alert to potential frostbite, since the first sign may be a loss of sensation. Unless heated, frostbite can kill body tissue. Keeping danger areas covered helps avoid the problem. A thin layer of Vaseline helps to protect lips and face. Penile frostbite may sound hilarious, but when it occurs, it is not a laughing matter. To prevent it, wear an extra pair of underwear.

Another rule is to wear items you can unzip or remove to carry. Even the best planning does not necessarily prepare you to face substantial temperature shifts. Clothing that seems barely warm enough at the start of a run may feel like a roaring furnace twenty minutes later. Zippers, sleeves that can be pushed up, and hats and gloves that come off easily are the key to comfortable winter running.

A final note on the direct effects of weather concerns the role of moisture. An uncomfortable rain at 50°F can be life-threatening at 32°F. An overlooked puddle that soaks your socks can lead to serious frostbite. Moisture destroys the insulation provided by air trapped between layers of clothing and also is a direct conduit for heat away from your body. A very thin nylon or water-resistant jacket can be an invaluable item in conserving your body heat.

Winter also brings special road problems. Hard, packed snow is a reasonable surface, but even though the rubber soles of running shoes provide relatively good traction, ice is hazardous. As road crews begin to clear streets, a new problem arises: competition for relatively scarce, passable roadway. The secret is not to win the confrontation with the automobile but to avoid it. Despite the best motivation in the world, cars maneuver poorly, stop slowly, and skid easily on winter streets. Be prepared to stop at intersections. If there is ever a time for defensive running, it is during the winter months.

Avoid rush hour. Wear bright clothing even during the day. Do not expect drivers to see you; the lower winter sun can impair vision even at midday, and snowstorms cut visibility drastically. Run *toward* traffic and be prepared to stop and step into an adjacent snowbank (it beats being knocked into one). Use extra caution because your headgear can muffle the sound of approaching cars.

Finally, a word about illnesses. Some people with asthma have cold-precipitated attacks, and if you notice wheezing or shortness of breath disproportionate to your level of training and speed, you may be having cold- or exercise-induced asthma. If the condition causes discomfort, seek medical attention because, for the most part, the problem is easily reversible or controllable.

People frequently ask about running with colds. In the absence of fever, some running, well within your limits, will probably not be harmful, and many people feel it helps them shake off the runny nose and other symptoms more quickly. Serious sinusitis, fever, muscle aches, and productive coughing are reasons not to run.

Frostbite, as mentioned before, is another medical problem, but it is preventable. It is uncommon in appropriately dressed runners, but it can occur as a result of moisture, inadequate clothing, or inappropriately long runs during which the body's ability to generate heat and pump blood to the extremities is simply exhausted. The fingers, toes, face, and ears are at greatest risk. Because numbness is an early symptom, the runner may not recognize the problem; if there is any question of impending frostbite, seek immediate shelter and warmth. Initially the skin will look white, but as rewarming occurs it becomes red, swollen, and may be painful. Rewarming should be accomplished with tepid water at temperatures between 100° and 110°F. Temperatures closer to 98.6°F can be used initially to reduce pain. Complete rewarming can take fifteen to twenty minutes. Emergency medical advice may be needed and is mandatory if the area remains cold and/or numb after rewarming.

Exhaustion in winter can be a serious problem, especially if you get stuck on a long (5–20 mile) run in an area with little traffic, are too tired to run and unable to generate sufficient body heat. Play by the rules, as if you were going cross-country skiing. If possible, run these distances with someone else, but be prepared to run single file on narrowed roads. Carry money, identification, and candy. Let someone know your route and approximate timetable and do not deviate from your plans.

Above all, use common sense. Plan shorter runs on cold days. Be prepared to alter your stride and slow your pace. Do not run in a heavy snowstorm, in icy rain, or on icy roads even if it means missing a day or two. A day off can be beneficial to tired muscles and joints, remember, and certainly is better than a month in a cast or worse. If you are a true running addict, find an indoor track or plan alternate activities such as cross-country skiing. If nothing else, an inclement day provides an excellent opportunity for extra stretching exercise and calisthenics.

Properly dressed and properly planned, outdoor running in the winter can be exhilarating. Traveling freely when cars are stranded, seeing the frozen countryside silhouetted in a low-lying, bright winter sun with blowing clouds of white steam the only hint of how cold it really is, and being covered by big flakes of white snow while comfortably warm are some of the special rewards of winter runs.

STRESS INJURIES

To improve fitness and performance, the body and its systems must be subjected to ever-increasing workloads. However, improved condition requires that the bodily systems be given sufficient opportunity to recover. Ignoring this second point causes the body and its systems to be thrown out of balance. The result is decreased performance, general fatigue, and in the extreme, stress injuries to the musculoskeletal system. Musculoskeletal problems, or "overuse syndromes," are caused by too many miles run too quickly; a biomechanical difficulty, usually in the foot or lower back; or a muscle imbalance of strength and/or lack of flexibility. Seek treatment for stress injuries from appropriate specialists: podiatrists treat foot injuries; physiotherapists, muscle problems; and orthopedic specialists, bone and leg-length discrepancies.

The foot area can suffer a wide variety of injuries with varying degrees of seriousness. Blisters, the most common foot malady, should be treated carefully by draining in a sterile way and applying a dressing of moleskin to avoid infection. Corns and calluses should be kept carefully trimmed; they can be temporarily removed with pumice stone. Injuries related to bones in the foot, such as stress fractures and bone bruises, with or without the eruption of blood between the bone and bone covering, should be given much rest and be checked by a specialist.

Use ice on painful injuries. Generally, a combination of ice, compression, and elevation will relieve pain. Ice has another medical virtue besides pain relief. It helps to stop bleeding—not only visible bleeding, but also bleeding that occurs under the skin, as when a shin is bruised. The black-and-blue discoloration is due to leakage of blood from torn blood vessels. An ice cube placed over the injured place constricts the blood vessels so there is less leakage until clotting takes place and thus reduces swelling, damage to the surrounding tissues, and pain, as well as discoloration.

Fill paper cups with water and store them in the freezer for that day when you need relief from pain. Peel the paper cup down as the ice melts against the injury.

Heat increases pain, swelling, and inflammation and usually is not a part of any immediate treatment for a running-related injury. When heat becomes a part of later treatment, moist heat is best. Hydrocollators are used for sore muscles.

ADVICE FOR THE INJURED RUNNER

John Cederholm of the Boston Athletic Association (BAA) offers a list of suggestions to follow if an injury occurs:

1. If it really hurts, stop running immediately. Take money on long training runs so you can take a bus or phone home for a ride.
2. Stop the inflammation; use ice and aspirin immediately.
3. Go to a hospital emergency ward. While waiting, try to get a diagnosis of your injury so that you don't waste time thinking your problem is something it isn't.
4. Once *you* know what the problem is, and if you need additional medical advice, consult a physician who is thoroughly familiar with runners and running injuries.
5. Because your injury probably resulted from overtraining, stay off your feet for one or two days and relax.
6. On day 3, start to run slowly. Resume normal training as pain subsides and as you regain confidence. Proper action during the first two days will result in a faster resumption of regular training and, hence, less loss of conditioning.

Remember: Follow your physician's advice and let your body tell you if the treatment is working. Each person is unique in terms of physical ability, general health, and recovery rate, so there has to be a great deal of flexibility in treatment of any running injury. Use common sense and listen to your body!

MOST COMMON INJURIES: CAUSES AND TREATMENT

Most running problems could be termed "overuse" or "stress injuries," which can be broadly characterized into tendon-muscle injuries, bone infractions, and injuries to joint surfaces. Of these categories, most important and numerous are those involving tendons.

Tendonitis

Tendonitis, the most common diagnosis made by a physician who sees many runners, is an inflammation of the tendon or of its thin, smooth lining, called the *tenosynovium.* The condition occurs as the result of repeated stress to a particular tendon, usually where it attaches to bone or crosses a body prominence. In runners, tendonitis characteristically strikes three areas: the Achilles tendon, the shins, and the knees.

In Achilles tendonitis, pain occurs either where the Achilles tendon attaches to the heel or just above that area. It may completely disable a runner because, every time he or she pushes off his or her foot, he or she has pain. Unfortunately, the primary treatment for tendonitis is rest and no running. For most runners, this remedy is unacceptable, and therefore, runners, trainers, and doctors have tried to figure out ways to run while in treatment for tendonitis. Among the measures of relieving Achilles tendonitis are elevation of the heel within the shoe to allow relaxation of the muscle tendon unit and decrease the stress on the tendon. Ice applied for ten to fifteen minutes to the tender area after running decreases the inflammatory response and pain. Oral anti-inflammatory agents ranging from aspirin to Phenylbutazone are helpful, too. Injection of steroids (cortisone preparations) into the tendon areas in active athletes is another treatment, but many physicians warn against using steroids. Injections may help but must be administered judiciously and, in runners, have limited usefulness. Surgery is rarely needed, but in severe cases it may be helpful. The procedure involves removing the diseased tenosynovium and any degenerated areas in the tendon and occasionally the bursa in front of and behind the Achilles tendon. Achilles tendonitis may require that a runner cease training for a period as long as six weeks. Shorter periods of time just do not seem to allow the condition to clear completely.

The term "shin splints" is an imprecise term used to describe a number of painful afflictions of the lower leg in runners. It probably should be restricted to pain in the lower leg on the medial aspect of the tibia, or what most runners' physicians feel is a tendonitis of the posterior tibial tendon. Local tenderness of the tibia over a three- or four-inch area is characteristic but may be confused with a stress fracture of the tibia, which causes more localized pain across the tibia, medially and laterally. By decreasing mileage, changing to a softer running surface, and using ice after activity, most runners can control shin splints while they gradually clear up. In some people, shin-splint pain is refractory and requires other treatment measures, such as oral anti-inflammatory agents, strengthening the dorsiflexion muscles of the foot, and stretching out the posterior calf muscles. Some trainers have success with strapping the leg to decrease the play of the posterior tibial tendon. Shin splints, along with other tendonitis problems, have a disturbing propensity for recurring. Rarely, the pain seems to be due to *ischemia* (lack of oxygen) of the muscles of the lower leg, which are caught in a tight anatomical compartment, and in these cases, surgical release of that compartment may be necessary.

When shin splints occur, and are confirmed by clinical diagnosis, treatment should consist of ice for a period of seven minutes, followed by ultrasound for a period of five minutes at 1.5. Following this procedure, it is recommended that a longitudinal arch strapping be applied and worn throughout each day until pain subsides. Best results are attained when treatment is done twice a day. Galvanic stimulation of the associated musculature may also minimize the pain and help to minimize edema. Anti-inflammatory agents, such as aspirin, do not appear to shorten the time lost from running. They do lessen discomfort, however, and permit near-normal ambulation.

Preventive maintenance consists of heat therapy (whirlpools at 108°F) prior to activity and cold therapy (ice packs for fifteen minutes or cold whirlpool for fifteen minutes) following activity. It is advisable, as stated earlier, to start a conditioning program consisting of total body exercises as well as specific exercises for the development of the frontal lower leg musculature, such as calf raises and toe curls. Proper warming up and cooling down are encouraged. A gradual increase in running mileage is recommended, as is a gradual transition from soft to hard surfaces. After running it is a good idea to do heel-cord or Achilles stretching to prevent shortening. Remember that prevention is the key to the treatment of shin splints, as is true with most overuse syndromes.

Two different types of tendonitis occur around the knee. One involves the large fascial band on the lateral side of the leg as it crosses over the bone of the knee joint to attach just below the knee. This iliotibial band is a major stabilizing structure on the lateral aspect of the knee, and the tendonitis pain is localized directly where the iliotibial band crosses the knee joint. Again, decreased mileage, ice, and anti-inflammatory agents are the usual treatments. As in all cases of tendonitis, the runner should reevaluate training routines. If the condition has come on after an increase in the training routine or, particularly, if the training ground has been changed from flat training to hills, the runner will have to back off. Rarely, a steroid injection may be used in iliotibial track tendonitis because in this location the injection is less of a problem. It is administered underneath the fascial band in the filmy tissues where the irritation has occurred.

Patellar tendonitis, sometimes called "jumper's knee," occurs where a patellar ligament attaches to the lower border of the kneecap. Sometimes this inflammation causes small degenerative tears within the tendon, which inhibits the tendon's capacity to repair itself. In this case, surgery to remove the degenerated portion may allow complete healing of the tendon.

In all cases of tendonitis, a runner's training routine will be compromised. Most often it is simply necessary to cut the mileage back each week. When pain is severe and the usual treatment does not suffice, the runner may have to discontinue training for as long as six weeks to allow everything to quiet down, and then begin training again slowly. This precaution does not always guarantee that the tendonitis will not recur. By varying their routines, decreasing mileage, and using some good common sense, however, most runners find that they're able to run with mild cases of tendonitis and to handle even severe cases.

Stress Fractures

Although we hear much about stress fractures in runners, the condition is less common than tendonitis, plantar fascitis, or chondromalacia. Stress fractures occur most commonly in the second and third metatarsals, but are also seen in the tibia, the lower part of the fibula, and even in the oscalcis. A stress fracture usually happens to people who have had relatively little running experience or people who have suddenly increased their weekly mileage. The pain starts insidiously and builds up; it is much worse when running. Runners who continue their training routines at this point risk getting the pain while walking. Localized tenderness and swelling are apparent right at the fracture site. X-rays taken within the first three weeks of symptoms will show nothing and the diagnosis may be missed. However, x-rays taken later will show a bony reaction, which means that the stress fracture is healing.

Treat runners with stress fractures by imposing a temporary, complete ban on running but allowing them to continue with normal walking activities and to maintain cardiovascular conditioning by bicycling and swimming. As long as there is point tenderness, the runner may not run. Once point tenderness has disappeared and the x-rays show complete healing, the runner then can resume training slowly and gradually. It is a mistake to go back to running until the point tenderness has completely disappeared.

Chondromalacia

Knee problems constitute the main source of injury for women runners. Twenty-eight percent of all women runners' athletic complaints concern the knee; principally, chondromalacia.

Runner's knee, or *chondromalacia,* is another imprecise term that refers to a variety of conditions. The condition seen most often is called "chondromalacia of the patella," which is a softening of the articular cartilage surface of the knee cap. It may be due to abnormal mechanics of the lower leg, ranging from an abnormal forward facing of the hip to knock knee or even pronation of the foot. All of these conditions increase lateral displacement of the knee cap and cause abnormal wear and tear on the patellar surface. Pain is usually felt deep in the knee or behind the knee cap. It is increased by running and by flexion of the knee.

Treatment for the condition varies with the cause. A pronated foot might need a medial arch support or a person with a knock-knee deformity could benefit from a foot orthosis to change the angulation of the foot at heel strike. Strengthening the anterior thigh muscles, or quadriceps, is effective because this muscle stabilizes the patella in its groove. This should be done isometrically, not by flexing the knee. Doing the exercises with the leg straight decreases stress on the knee cap. Regular doses of aspirin may be needed to relieve pain and inflammation of chondromalacia. The condition responds poorly to steroid injections of the knee and they should not be used. Runners with chondromalacia often can continue training routines at a decreased level. They should avoid running on hilly courses, however, and particularly going downhill, and training routines should be modified accordingly.

Some people with severe chondromalacia simply may not be able to run. Surgery is a possibility. Surgery usually consists of trying to realign the patella mechanism so the knee cap stays within its groove, but it is the last resort for a runner. However, if pain persists and particularly if there is swelling, an arthroscopic examination of the knee joint would reveal the damage to the back side of the patella. If there is significant damage, then a realignment procedure is in order.

Plantar Fasciitis

One other difficult problem is pain in the sole of the foot near the heel bone. This is usually the result of an inflamation of the plantar fascia where it attaches to the heel bone. Sometimes, it may be caused by irritation of a small nerve in the same area. Direct tenderness over the plantar fascia is a tip to the diagnosis. Most people complain of pain upon taking the first thirty or forty steps in the morning or after they have been sitting for a while. They usually have pain at the beginning of a run and then feel better for a while but gradually start to have increased pain after three or four miles.

Icing after running is helpful for this condition and done faithfully may allow people to continue to run while nature gradually cures the problem. Various types of foot orthoses have been prescribed, but I find that suppporting the plantar fascia with a soft orthosis is of more help than trying to cushion the heel. Sometimes, however, a heel cup does bring relief. Oral anti-inflammatory medications may be quite helpful and so, occasionally, is a steroid injection. Plantar fasciitis is particularly frustrating because every time the runner lands on his or her foot, the pain increases. Usually judicious icing, anti-inflammatory agents, a proper orthosis and decreasing mileage allow a runner to continue to be on the road. Only rarely is it necessary to operate and release the plantar fascia.

The appearance of a heel spur on an x-ray means nothing. The spur is not the cause of pain but simply an indication of the location of the plantar fascia attachment. Many people have heel spurs without pain, and many people with plantar fasciitis do not have heel spurs.

OTHER MEDICAL PROBLEMS

There are other problems of a medical nature that runners may experience. One is "jogger's kidney," a pseudo disease caused by athletic activity in which laboratory tests show abnormal amounts of protein, red blood cells and other substances in the runner's urine. This turns out to be a transient problem brought on by prolonged exercise of an hour or more at a time. Jogger's kidney usually lasts about two days. The condition is probably triggered by the fact that part of the blood that would normally be sent to the kidneys for cleaning is sent to working muscles during running. This switch confuses the kidney function and causes proteins and other elements to end up in the urine. The condition resembles the serious kidney disease nephritis.

Sciatica, or back pain, causes suffering for many runners. Sciatica is pain from your back through your buttocks and posterior leg, sometimes to the toes. It is often accompanied by numbness and tingling. All these problems frequently are linked to muscular weakness and especially to flabby stomach muscles.

The best exercise for combatting weak stomach muscles is sit-ups. Sit-ups should be done with the hips and knees bent to flatten out the back and relax the hip flexors. This approach takes the strain off the back and makes the abdominal muscles work hard.

HELPFUL HINTS: STANDARD TREATMENT PROCEDURE FOR RUNNING INJURIES

First day:

1. Injury recognition (history, inspection, limitation)
2. Apply cold, wet compression and ice; elevate the area
3. If you cannot move normally, restrict with sling, splint, crutches; refer to M.D.

Second day (A.M. and P.M.):

1. X-ray if fracture suspected; refer to M.D.
2. If swelling persists, continue first-day treatment
3 If not swollen:

    a.   Apply hot, moist heat packs for twenty minutes
    b.   Lightly massage (around area) and lightly exercise
    c.   Apply analgesic packs or Ben-Gay

Third day and thereafter:

1. Whirlpool at 98°–100° F for twenty minutes and/or ultrasound
2. Massage—light exercise increasing gradually to participation
3. Protect area with supportive taping or wrapping

Muscle strain results when some of the muscle fibers pull apart and cause a certain amount of bleeding in the muscle. The purpose of conditioning is to strengthen muscles enough so that they will not come apart.

Most people go into running for reasons different from people who choose other sports. They do it for the competition and for the physical training. They physically feel better, and that is why they run, so the injuries they complain about are much different, too. Runners are much more conscious of every little ache and pain. They run for their bodies, so they are more conscious of their bodies.

No one should ignore pain, because some pain does indicate that the body has been overstressed; however, some of the aches and pains of running just have to be tolerated until the condition of the muscles improves. Limbering the joints and loosening the muscles with stretching exercises before and after running is recommended. Beginners must be careful not to overstretch their muscles and joints. Stretching, like conditioning, should be slow and accomplished gradually. You should not push past the limits of the muscles and joints.

There are guidelines that runners can use to evaluate pain. Duration is the key to the significance of a particular pain. Medical attention is necessary when the beginning runner experiences one or a combination of the following symptoms: redness, swelling, pain, or heat. Any pain that starts during the run and persists for more than three or four days requires professional attention.

A stress fracture is not just one sudden crack in the bone. It stems from repeated stress over a long period of time. Prolonged stress eventually wears down the bone in a particular spot. With shin splints, the anterio muscle coming over the tibia (the muscle that helps you flex your foot) is very strained and running over the bone. Part of it has separated from the bone, and the muscles continue to pull away from their origin. Shin splints are almost always a result of not having the muscles up to par. People who get shin splints are usually those who increase their mileage too fast or who increase their mileage and do hills at the same time. They are also a result of tight calf muscles, an imbalance between the calf muscles and the shin muscles that allows one muscle to overpower the other. They are one reason why stretching is important.

Knee-cap problems are also more common in a beginning runner and often come from a malalignment of the knee cap. Orthoses can help some knee problems because they change the position of the foot. Strengthening the quadriceps can also alleviate certain knee problems, as these are the muscles that surround and support the knee.

8

RACING STRATEGY

There's no substitute for racing experience. If you haven't yet raced, reading this chapter won't turn you into a seasoned competitor, no matter how hard you study it. What the principles outlined below *will* do is to help you make the most efficient use of the hard training you've been doing to get in racing shape. No matter how fit you are, making the wrong moves in a race will squander your physical reserves and make you run ultimately slower than you actually can.

You should also think of the points below as guidelines for observations during your races. If you keep the principles in mind while competing, you'll suddenly find yourself thinking, "Ah-ha, that's what he meant!" when you actually encounter the situations you've been studying.

To help yourself develop as a racer, make detailed notes of your race in your training diary, and then study them the day after the race. Even professional runners are often too wound up, or worn out, after the race to assess accurately what they did right and what they did wrong. Next to your shoes, your training diary is the single most valuable tool you have. Use it; the scientific runner will always beat the undisciplined one.

YOUR FIRST RACE: THE TIME DOESN'T MATTER

Regardless of the distance of your first race, you should have two strategic goals in mind for it: (1) to finish, and (2) to enjoy yourself.

These goals are more important than *any* others as far as your first race is concerned. This is because a positive mental and emotional attitude is even more important to racing success than is excellent physical conditioning. (See Chapter 6—Mental/Emotional Aspects of Running.) Your first race has a profound effect on how you will come to think of competitive running. If it's a negative experience, you're not too likely to be psyched up at your next race; more likely, you'll be unconsciously tense and cringing.

A serious athlete never enters a race he or she is not completely confident he or she has the training to finish. *The only exception to this rule is your first race*. There's a huge difference between believing something at the intellectual level and *knowing* it at the emotionally integrated level. Your first race will be the only one you'll have to summarize with the reply, "I finished!" From the second race on, you'll be answering the question with your time and finishing place. People who constantly "race" only to finish do not think of themselves as athletes; and the difference between a jogger and a runner has nothing to do with speed. It has to do with whether or not you think of yourself as an athlete.

THINK TANK: STRATEGIC BASICS

1. *Start:* Get away quickly and assume your normal running stride as soon as possible. That first mile hurts everyone.
2. *Pace:* From proper practice sessions, each individual should have some knowledge of proper pace. To be on the safe side, wear a wrist stopwatch. It's not uncommon for a race course to have the mile markers in the wrong spot. It's also not uncommon to be given inaccurate split times by roadside volunteers. A wrist stopwatch not only gives you your time for the race as soon as you cross the finish line, it also gives you an objective indication of how far you've come and how far you've left to go. Distribution of energy at proper, pre-planned tempo is the plan.
3. *Knowledge of opponents:* The athlete becomes aware of oppo-

nents' strengths and weaknesses by noting how they run a race. Of course, they're also checking *you* out—so try to be prepared with new moves in the next race. Not only will this throw your opposition off guard, it will make you a more versatile, well-rounded athlete.

4. *Hill running:* Think positively about running hills (and see the section on hill running, below). Don't become intimidated instead. When you come to a hill, think to yourself, "Here's my chance to blow this guy/gal away." Hills are like the first mile of a race: everybody hurts, but those who don't let the hurting get them down go on to become winners.

5. *Knowledge of the course:* Hills are less of an emotional upset if you know exactly when to expect them. Few things are more demoralizing then suddenly finding out the course ends with an uphill (as Falmouth does). The same thing goes for any other unexpected course quirks, such as an unusually narrow

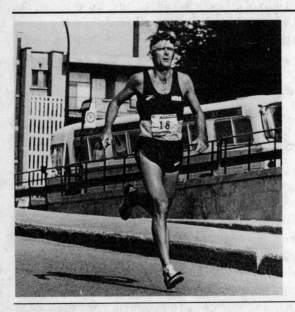

A runner on a downhill section of the Montreal Marathon shows good downhill form; notice that his leading foot falls directly beneath his center of gravity. (Photograph courtesy of George J. Marcelonis)

section that precludes passing, a surprise dirt-and-rocks stretch on an otherwise paved road, a hulking guard dog on somebody's lawn adjacent to the route. Make every attempt to go over the course a day prior to competition. Warm up over the first and last miles, if the course is a loop, on race day. If the race is point-to-point and the start and finish areas are prohibitively far apart, it's more desirable to know the lay of the land at the end of the course (where you'll be sagging) than at the start (where you'll be fresh and strong).

6. *Group running:* It's crowded out there, sometimes. Always practice this skill with companions in workouts, so you'll know how to avoid tripping over others, and how to keep them from boxing you in.

7. *Finish:* All distance runners become sprinters. Always presume there's somebody right at your elbow when the finish line comes up; in a huge race, there probably *will* be one or more people you didn't see before closing in on you. Each week incorporate sprint pick-ups in your training program on the run. Make a strong effort not to let down either your physical or mental concentration until *after* you've crossed the line—and make sure you know *exactly* where the finish line is. (Is it that chalk mark on the ground, the "Finish Line" banner several feet in front of it, or where that guy with the stopwatch is standing? If you don't know *for sure,* keep your kick until you're actually in the finish chute.)

8. *Review results:* How effective were the tactics employed during the competition? Was there any quick pick-up by an opponent at various points? Poor hill running, slow start? Analysis of these performance factors will improve your racing techniques.

RACING STRATEGY I:
THE 6-MILE OR 10-KILOMETER RACE

1. Take the 2 days before the race to evaluate what you did in the 2 *trial* races included in the training schedule. Did you go out too fast? Too slow? Not have anything left for a sprint at the finish? Get discouraged by a hill? We learn more from our

mistakes than from our successes. By evaluating your trial runs, you guarantee yourself success in THE BIG ONE.

2. Use the speed you've developed from your pick-ups and hill running in the first 1½ miles. It should be one sustained pick-up. *Don't* slow down after the 1-mile split. Fight hard against the natural tendency to back off your mental concentration when you hear your 1-mile time. Whatever you do, don't be shocked if the 1-mile split's much faster than you'd intended. If you feel comfortable, you've just learned you're a lot faster than you thought. *Don't* start to worry about being able to finish at this pace. You already know you can finish. It's the bozos who freak when they hear a fast first-mile split; it's the real runners who are encouraged by such a thing, and press on just as hard.

3. Settle into a strong, steady pace at 1½ miles; 85 percent of all runners in the race will have settled into their race pace by this point. Waiting until 1½ miles before settling into race pace puts you in the second of four competitive groups (elite runners, hard-core runners, those who *should* be hard-core runners, and the plodders). Only the elite athletes should keep up his or her sprint beyond 1½ miles in a 6-miler or 10K.

4. The position you hold at 2 miles will be, within 3 places up or down, the position in which you'll finish the race, unless something goes drastically wrong. Because you have trained properly, nothing will go drastically wrong. It's a matter of hanging on from here on in; take strength from how far up in the field you are, and how well you're going to finish in your first BIG race!

5. Hold race pace until the 4-mile mark. It's getting really tough for everybody now. Every person you see in front of you is hurting every bit as much as you are, maybe more. *Now* use your upper-body strength to pick up the pace. Not very many people do much passing after 2 miles in a 10K road race, but there's no reason at all *you* can't be one of the strong ones who does pass in the later stages. Think how depressing it must be to your competition to have you surge by them when they're dragging their tails in exhaustion. No matter how fagged-out *you* may really be, 99 percent of the people you pass will think you're a lot fresher than they are, and let you go without a fight.

6. The finish line's just ahead. Don't relax your concentration or effort, but keep as loose as possible. Stay cool and ready for anything, such as the hero who comes up on you suddenly at a sub-4 pace. *Don't forget to stop your watch when you cross the line.* Knowing your time will give you an immediate, well-deserved reward for your hard race and may very well help settle any foul-ups that sometimes happen in official results.

7. Take a proper warm-down. You'll be able to boogie a lot longer at the post-race party if you do. You'll also be able to get back into normal training a lot sooner if you do. Jog a mile or so, do your complete stretching routine, and lie on your back with your feet elevated over your head for 4–5 minutes. While doing this, *evaluate* your race, and plan changes in your training to compensate for deficiencies that showed up. (Did you "die" at the end of the race? You need to work on your endurance. A lot of people passed you on the long downhill? You need to work on your hill technique.)

RACING STRATEGY II: THE 10-MILE OR 15-KILOMETER RACE

1. Employ the same strategy as for the 6-mile or 10K race up to the 5-mile mark. Do a hard 1-minute pick-up at 5 miles; most seasoned competitors will put in a surge around this point to see if they can jockey into a higher position. (The longer the race, the more strategy there is involved.)

2. Use the space from 6 to 7 miles to recover from your hard pick-up. Be careful not to let yourself "die" during this interval, though. When you're recovering during the course of an actual race, it doesn't mean that you slow down very much; instead, it means you *relax*. A major relaxation in intense physical and concentrative effort translates into a relatively minor reduction in speed if the athlete is in proper condition.

3. From 7 miles on to the finish, concentrate on holding your form and driving to the end. Most people are slowing down now, and it's from mental fatigue as much as from physical exhaustion. Good running form is more a result of intellectual concentration than it is a result of physical conditioning. The

better your form, the more efficiently you will run and use your remaining energy. A small lapse in mental effort therefore means a significant reduction in running efficiency; hence, in running speed. Fight against the fatigue, and let it work against your opponents. Don't forget to use your upper-body strength to help pull you through the last few miles. Too many distance runners forget their arms are actually a pair of auxiliary legs!

4. Use the same end-of-race procedures as outlined above for shorter races.

RACING STRATEGY III: THE MARATHON

1. Your last workout is 12 days before the race (see marathon training schedule). This gives you plenty of time to recover and be properly rested on THE BIG DAY.

2. The hardest instruction to follow in marathon racing strategy has nothing to do with the actual race itself. The instruction is to *relax during the week before the race.* Expect to feel edgy now. Because you're not doing hard workouts, your body has energy to spare. The impending race is also, naturally, making you nervous. This is perfectly normal. *Don't* start thinking you're losing your conditioning. Remind yourself of 2 things: (1) *rest is part of training,* and (2) there's *nothing* you can do the week before any sort of race to help yourself win it, but there's *plenty* you can do to yourself the week before a race to help yourself *lose* it. If you start feeling edgy, do things around the house and take your mind off working out on the roads. Very few people rest enough the week before the race. Let one of the smart ones be *you.*

3. Eat enough just to stay alive until 1½ days before the race. You need rest, but you don't need added weight the week before any race. Because you're resting, you need fewer calories than when training hard. Do anything to take your mind off your nervousness *other than* stuffing your face.

4. When you do start to load up on food, be guided by common sense, not by apparent running tradition. If the athlete does

not normally eat highly spiced foods, he or she should avoid chowing down on a huge plate of garlic-and-pepper pasta at Mama Inferno's Restaurant. Eat only foods you know you can digest easily.

5. Remember to take a 15-minute walk after the pre-race meal (16 hours before the race) to help digestion and limber up muscles.

6. The Wall is not what marthoners hit when their glycogen is depleted. The Wall is what marathoners climb the night before the big race. Make contingency plans to eliminate the impact of a wakeful pre-race night. First, get an excellent sleep *two* nights before the race. A well-trained athlete can compensate for poor sleep the night immediately before a race if he or she is fundamentally well-rested two days before. Second, keep the bedroom cool and well-ventilated. A hot, stuffy room is a surer "cure" for sleep than a brass band playing next door.

7. Pack your equipment and look over your paraphernalia checklist carefully. Be prepared for all types of weather. Make sure you have a thermos bottle filled with water.

8. Drink fluid replacement drinks (e.g., ERG) with meals the day before the race, but drink water on race day. Keep the water at room temperature, not cold. Cold water can hit the athlete's warm stomach and cause cramping.

9. It is very important to arrive at the start location at least one hour before time. You must check in for a pre-race physical, receive your number, relieve yourself. Drink some water from your thermos.

10. Go to the starting line and position yourself with athletes of comparable ability. Find 3 other people who want to run the same time that you do, and run together with them as a team. Don't retreat to the back line unless you belong there. At the final countdown to the starting gun, set your watch so you will have proper timing en route. *Remember:* the splits you hear called to you during the first 3 miles of a major (more than 3,000 runners) marathon will not be an accurate index of your performance because of all the congestion. Don't expect to be able to settle on a good pace for yourself until 4 to 6 miles into the competition.

12. If you're a highly competitive athlete and deserve to start

from the front of the pack, treat the start of a marathon the way you treat the start of a shorter race: get out fast for the first 1½ miles. If you're a sub-elite athlete, resign yourself to the congestion (*and remember that the congestion will be even worse if you position too far toward the front*) and start picking it up between 4 and 6 miles, when the crowd thins out. Broken-field running is fine for halfbacks, stupid for marathoners, who need every iota of energy they can preserve.

13. The elite athlete will hold his or her initial pick-up until 6 miles into the marathon. The above-average runner will hold the pick-up for about 3 miles. Athletes of all levels of ability should strive for an even pace between 6 and 20 miles.

14. Most serious athletes make a move at about 15 kilometers or 10 miles. Ideally, you've selected a group of marathon veterans to run with. They're going to move at this point, although it will not (or should not) be like an end-of-race sprint. You must be prepared to move with your group.

15. Remember to take a drink at each water station, even if you must slow to a jog to get that 3 ounces of fluid into your body. If possible, have friends on the course with a plastic water bottle or ice cubes. It's a bonus you won't regret.

16. At the halfway point (13.1 miles) you'll make another pick-up like the one at around 10 miles, or 15 kilometers. Your half-point split should be within 1½ minutes of the pace necessary to make your target finishing time. If your split is too fast, you really can't expect to back off and recoup the losses you've laid on your body. If you have gone out unwisely fast, cut your losses and fall back to a slower goal-time, and run at a much slower pace. Console yourself with the knowledge you'll never go out too fast again.

17. What you feel at 20 miles into the marathon is what you felt at around 17 or 18 miles in your 20-mile training runs; therefore, do what you did in your training at that point. Relax all over, take turns setting the pace with your partners. Shake your arms to get any tension out of them, and keep your hands loose and your breathing rhythmic.

18. An unprepared runner worries about "the Wall" at 20 miles. For you, the serious athlete, there is no "Wall," but there is the "Twilight Zone" of the marathon that begins about 23 miles and lasts through to the finish. *Everybody* who can run

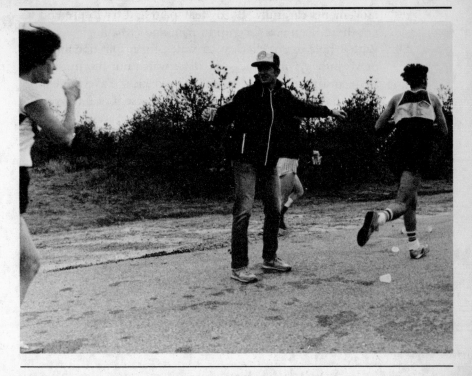

Practice taking fluids so you can keep on racing. Make sure it's water in the cup you take, and not a soft drink! (Photograph by Bill Boyle)

in the top half of the pack is hurting at this point, from the winner on down. This is when the mind takes over from the body. The willpower that motivated your hard, often inconvenient, training for the last eight months will pull you through. Your mind has to keep your arms (especially vital in this last stage of the race) and legs pumping. You only have 15 to 18 minutes of running left. You *know* you can run for 18 minutes on the worst possible day of your life; therefore, you now *know* you will finish *on schedule.*

19. Your mind is so important to you at this stage that you must not let your imagination short-circuit it. The worst possible mistake you could make now is to try to imagine away your discomfort. Accept it; monitor all your body's systems and

movements carefully. Bozos fear pain and try to pretend it's not there. Runners face up to pain and *break* it.

20. With 1 mile to go, check your watch for inspiration and then move into a 1-mile pick-up. *Don't* wait until the finish is in sight and then let loose with a torrid kick. Take the energy from that hundred-yard kick and disperse it evenly over the last mile. Your time will be much faster that way.
21. Stop your watch when crossing the line and give yourself the reward you've earned: an excellent marathon time.

You should train at half-load for seven days and then add two miles a day until you get back to your training average. There is a tendency for people to want to race after a good performance. Three weeks after a marathon, you may run a 6-to 10-mile race. Do not run a marathon more often than every three to four months, regardless of what you may see elite athletes doing. You should run the other races to gain speed and strength.

RACING TIP: RUNNING DOWN HILLS

Running uphill is a science, but running downhill is an art. You've learned how to run uphill properly by incorporating hill workouts into your weekly training; but many people can run down hills forever and not get the knack of how to do it well. Conversely, there are some who get the downhill "feel" from their very first attempt.

To run well uphill requires sheer strength. To run well downhill demands almost no strength at all, but two other things that may be even harder to come by: an excellent sense of balance and sheer courage. In other words, to run well downhill means to have total confidence in yourself.

You know that to run well uphill you must shorten your stride, pull *hard* with your arms, make a strong effort to keep your shoulders and the muscles between your shoulder blades loose and relaxed, and bend forward not from the waist but from the *small of the back*. (Running uphill puts tremendous strain on your back muscles; do bent-knee sit-ups regularly to strengthen your girdle muscles and prevent injuries from muscle imbalances.) When you are in the proper posture for running uphill, you will find your gaze falls about six feet directly in front of you—and that's with your neck totally perpendicular with your torso. You're not bending your head down, you're bending your upper body more parallel with the incline of the hill. If you have strong quadriceps muscles, you'll climb that hill like crazy. If your quads aren't strong, doing your weekly hill repeats will make them so.

To run downhill well requires a combination of proper form and proper mental attitude. (By the way, don't wait for a mountainous hill before you shift from your flat-running posture to the proper hill-running posture. Treat *every* incline as a hill. Most runners, even competitive ones, have terrible form. Don't be one of them.) To run downhill well, you have to want to run downhill well with a passion; just as, to truly run fast, you must *want* to do so passionately. Running well downhill confers three major benefits to the athlete: (1) it's enormously fun; (2) it allows you to blow your competition into the weeds (if you run the hill hard); (3) it permits you to pace with your competition while catching a big rest as they struggle along (if you run the hill easy). That summarizes the proper mental attitude.

The best way to understand the proper downhill running form is by studying the great 100-meter runners. Notice how far over they lean when they come off the blocks—think of Houston McTear! McTear says that if he didn't come off the line as fast as he does (and he's probably the world's fastest *thing* up to 60 yards), he would fall face-down. Take a lesson from that: Think of running downhill as constantly starting to fall butt-over-teakettle and constantly catching yourself. Your accelerative force is Mother Gravity, on a down hill. You can run much faster than your muscles will take you. The only things that limit your speed, then, are (1) how much pounding your skeleton can take (and the more efficient your form, the more stress you keep *off* your body), and (2) how far over you are willing to lean when running downhill.

To be blunt, the ideal would be for you to take a spill at least once in your training. The only precise way to know your limits is to press beyond them occasionally.

What kind of downhill stride should you have? The runners with the best form on uphills, downhills, and flats are those who run unconsciously (e.g., Toshihiko Seko). Don't worry about where your foot falls. Let nature take care of that. Just have it fall where it always should, regardless of the terrain you're running: directly beneath your center of gravity. If your feet always fall right under your center of gravity, you know you have the perfect stride for the conditions.

The way you use your arms in running downhill depends on how mature a downhill athlete you are. You will go through two stages here. First, when learning your way down the hills, hold your arms out almost like wings. This will give you added stability, and confidence. Then, when your confidence reaches the point it must, *stop thinking about what to do with your arms.* Relax. *If* you've good basic arm carriage (a big "if"), just do what comes naturally. If you don't have good arm carriage already, keep your hands and forearm muscles very relaxed, drive very slightly with your shoulder (deltoid) muscles, and don't even let your arms swing from side to side—ideally, you will have trained your arms (through running itself, and through free weight workouts) to swing always parallel with your legs, with almost no lateral motion. Lateral arm motion throws you off-balance—the last thing you need in downhill running—and wastes energy as you constantly have to correct your posture and direction of travel. This is an apparently subtle waste of energy until you've experienced the right way to do it. Finally, let your arms hang down around the bottom of your rib cage. Don't hold them up like you think somebody's going to throw a punch at you, and don't ever let them fall below the level of your hipbones (unless it is to shake them briefly to loosen your arms up during a race or workout).

Running downhill punishes the body severely, no matter how little you weigh and how good you are at it. You should not practice it too much. Because running downhill is almost completely a mental, not a physical, skill, you will never lose it once you have the knack for it.

9

WHAT KIND OF RUNNER DO YOU WANT TO BE?

This book is for two types of runners, the one who wants to train to be able to race and the one who wants to train to become fitter and healthier. Sometimes these two different runners occupy the same althlete's body and fight over control of his/her heart and mind. More often, the runner finds his or her values shifting gradually back and forth between those exemplified by these two different archetypes, a result of growing athletic experience (or sometimes the shocking result of an injury or unexpected race victory). We think that the complete runner embraces the values of both the racer and the fitness-and-health enthusiast. The distinction we make between these two types of runners in this book when giving training guidelines is somewhat artificial, but it is also practical.

How to Use the Training Guidelines

You'll notice that our training schedules in Part II are numbered sequentially, starting with Stage 1. The Stage 1 training schedule is for someone who has never run a step and wants to start a running program. You may already be a fit runner as you read this for the first time. There is no need, then, for you to start at Stage 1. Look through the different training schedules until you find one that matches your present level of running. You may find that you will be starting in on one of the later weeks of one of the training programs. If you've been running about 25 miles a week on a 5-day schedule of your own, for example, you'd start training with week 8 to 9 of the Basic Fitness Program, which is Stage 2F.

You of course need not "run" through the entire book. When you reach a fitness level that satisfies you, just keep repeating the training for that week, or perhaps keep cycling through the week and the one that precedes it. You can then move on to the more intense training we've outlined any time you may later decide to.

It may happen that you are constrained from following your normal training schedule. When more urgent matters demand you give up some of your running time, turn to Stage 5, the Contingency Maintenance Program. This schedule will help you maintain your fitness temporarily while you devote the attention necessary to your more important priorities.

You'll notice that the running training schedules above Stage 1 all have a suffix of either *F* or *R*. The letter *F* indicates a training schedule for the health-and-fitness runner, while *R* indicates a schedule for the racer. Anyone who has never before run starts at Stage 1, whether he or she wants to race or to run for fitness.

We have interspersed the F and R schedules because you, as a complete runner, will want to know about all aspects of training as a runner. We felt that to divide the F and R schedules into two different sections in the Training Schedules part of this book would imply that they are for two totally different types of athlete. Not so. As we've already said, distinctions between the racer and the health-and-fitness enthusiast are artificial. We'd like now to explain what differences there are between these two types of running, to help you understand the distinctions we have structured into the training we provide.

The Different Types of Running

At the start of a beginning runner's training, there is no behavioral distinction between the racer and the fitness runner. The fitter the racer, the more likely he or she is to win races. But there are significant differences between the attitudes of the racer and the fitness runner from the very first day of training. (We should point out, though, that one of the world's most common stories concerns the overweight person who started jogging to lose weight, discovered he or she had talent as a competitor, and shifted over from the mentality of the fitness runner to that of the racer.) These differences in attitudes soon enough result in differences in behavior, training, and global cumulative stress.

Truly competitive racers run beyond the point of diminishing returns for achieving fitness—sometimes, way beyond it. Many feel this kind of training is necessary when world-class races are won or lost by hundredths of a second. The point is debatable. What is indisputable is that such training is not healthy. If often results in injury. It usually results in emotional stress. It always overdevelops some parts of the body in relation to other parts. The racer is *dedicated* in the precise definition of the word—dedicated both as a personality and as a physical machine. His or her goal is not good health, nor even fitness as such. It is to win races.

Dr. Stan James, an orthopedic surgeon who has repaired many world-class runners, once commented about racers: "I feel that there are a lot of elite athletes training beyond the maximum benefits that they really want. There's a curve with diminishing returns. A lot of them could get by with less training and still maximize their potential. The philosophy seems to be: 'How far can I carry my training without getting injured?' *My* attitude is: 'How little can you do and still maximize your performance, so you don't even come close to developing an illness or injury?' "

Many coaches and elite runners believe that the hobbyist racers are even worse than the world-class gals and guys in terms of whipping themselves! The schedules we offer for racers in this book are in line with Dr. James's attitude of doing as little work as necessary to bring out your best. But many racers are self-coached, or coached with more enthusiasm than sense. They've been injured, disillusioned, burned-out. And so the one-time racer, who may have started jogging just to lose some weight, gives up racing but wants to keep running, and turns into a fitness runner. This is a typical example of what we mean by a runner's values tending to shift back and forth between racing and running for health and fitness.

It is a sad thing to feel forced to do something because another thing you preferred to do did not work out as you'd hoped. It's particularly sad when the apparent failure resulted from misinformation or excessive zeal, instead of lack of talent, desire, or determination. If you are a former racer like the kind we just described, run for fitness and maintain—we hope, restore—your enthusiasm, fit-

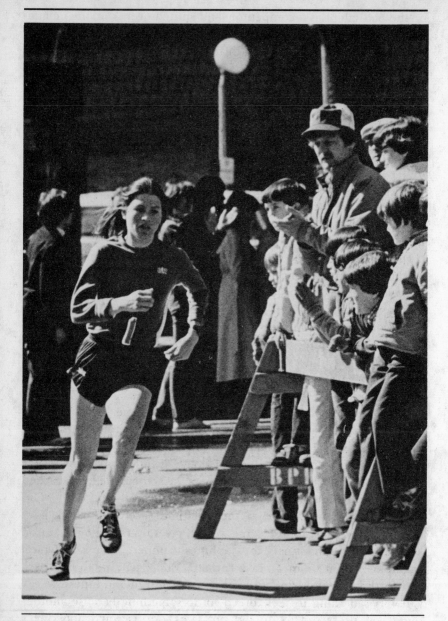

*Patti Catalano demonstrates good running form rounding a corner.
(Photograph by Bill Boyle)*

ness, and self-confidence. And, if you some day again want to race, try it with our help.

The overwhelming majority of *you* runners are running for health and fitness. You were always the backbone of the running boom. You do not run to excess. Running may not even be your primary means of exercise. It's likely you play other sports or follow other structured sorts of workouts, such as swimming, bicycling, skiing, or weight lifting. There's a good chance your running is as much for mental health and fitness as it is for physical benefits. Indeed, because of the emotional pleasure you take from running, it probably doesn't matter to you very much what physical benefits the sport may offer.

The health-and-fitness runner is motivated by the goal of having fun—fun in running, and fun as a result of running. The racer is motivated by the goal of doing well in, or winning, races—a very specific type of fun. The racer brings to running the intensity that comes from narrow focus of goal and effort. The health-and-fitness runner (particularly those with Type A personalities) is as determined as the racer, but determined to have fun in a much broader sense. It has become more popular to engage in a wide variety of athletics since the first edition of *Improving Your Running* appeared. Seeking new ways of having fun, the fitness runner has moved on to embrace other sports as part of his or her athletics. That is why the fitness running schedules we provide require fewer days of running per week than do the racing schedules. That is also why we have expanded our advice about supplementary strength-building techniques for runners. Fitness runners have more interest in other sports than they did during the height of the running boom.

Racers also have more interest in alternative forms of exercise than they did a few years ago. This is the result of eager racers becoming injured as a result of their athletics and having to use other exercises as a way to maintain their fitness, and sometimes as therapy, for their injuries. Interest in exercise that supplements running is a development among both racers and runners over the past seven years or so. It is a parallel development that helps demonstrate our belief that there is little difference between the racer and the runner. The main difference between them concerns attitudes and goals.

Only you can decide what kind of runner you want to be. The kind you want to be today may not be the kind you want to be two years from now. We'd be surprised if it were. Your training needs alone will change as a result of athletics becoming increasingly ingrained in your life. Your nutritional and recuperative needs will surely be different after two more years of training than they are today, even if you are already an advanced athlete. As a person, you will have two more years of emotional maturity. We'd be very surprised if the runner you want to be in two years is the same as the runner you want to be this afternoon. That is good. Change is one of the few constants in nature. The goal of athletic training of any sort is to become healthier, fitter, and have more fun by means harmonious with natural law. Decide what you want from running, and that will determine what kind of runner you want to be. Then get out and run, happy with your decision. Perhaps the biggest running secret of all is that a light heart makes for easy running. No matter how much advice we give you in this book, only you can make your heart light.

Go run.

Part II

TRAINING SCHEDULES

10

WORKOUTS FOR YOUNGSTERS

The following training programs are intended for boys and girls in the sixth, seventh, or eighth grades. Youngsters in the ninth grade and up may follow the Walk-Jog-Run or Fun Run training programs found in Chapters 12 and 14.

Warning: It is very inadvisable to start a child on a formal training program in any one sport before the sixth grade. Premature concentration in any athletic discipline robs the child of enjoying a wide variety of sports, an enjoyment that pays big dividends later in life when the person becomes a spectator at, or participant in, different types of athletics. Further, although mature athletes must concentrate on their sport-specialty in order to become truly excellent, we find time and again that the most outstanding sports specialists had a strong multisport background before deciding on their specialty. Most athletes who start young in a structured, formal training program grow bored of the sport by their early teen years. Parents should encourage their children to run only as the child's natural inclinations make him or her want to run.

None of this means that this is the only suitable chapter in this book for youngsters' eyes. The sections on proper warm-up and warm-down, nutrition, and correct running posture will also be interesting to the young runner—especially if he or she decides to read them on his or her own. Remember, nobody likes a pushy parent—least of all that parent's child.

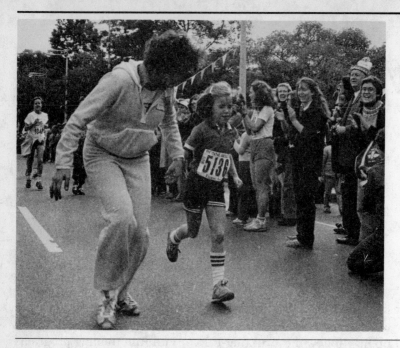

If your children want to run, by all means take an interest, but do not push them to race or compete. This little girl's happy smile indicates she has a supportive parent or friend. (Photograph courtesy of George J. Marcelonis)

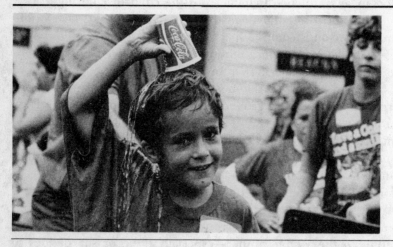

Children need to take care to cool off during a race just as much as adults do. (Photograph courtesy of George J. Marcelonis)

PROGRAM PROCEDURES: YOUNGSTERS

SIXTH GRADE: WEEK 1

	Jog	Walk	Jog	Walk	Comments
Day 1					
Track*	½ mile	¾ mile	½ mile	½ mile	
Time	6 minutes	15 minutes	6 minutes	10 minutes	
Day 2					
Track	½ mile	¾ mile	½ mile	½ mile	
Time	6 minutes	15 minutes	6 minutes	10 minutes	
Day 3	Day off				
Day 4					
Track	¾ mile	½ mile			
Time	9 minutes	10 minutes			
Day 5					
Track	¾ mile	½ mile			
Time	9 minutes	10 minutes			
Day 6	Day off				
Day 7					
Track	Mile	¾ mile			
Time	12 minutes	15 minutes			

*Use running track or measured distance. On days off, practice other sports.

There's A DOG on My Favorite Training Route!

So what? If you remain calm, he probably will, too—unless you're trepassing on his territory, which you should not. ("His territory" means the spot on which he sleeps. Dog owners who think their pet is "territorial" because he bites anybody he sees in the park where he's walked every day know nothing at all about animal territoriality. They don't have a territorial dog; they have a vicious dog.)

PROGRAM PROCEDURES: YOUNGSTERS

SIXTH GRADE: WEEK 2

	Jog	Walk	Jog	Walk	Comments
Day 1					
Track	½ mile	¾ mile	½ mile	½ mile	
Time	6 minutes	15 minutes	6 minutes	10 minutes	
Day 2					
Track	½ mile	¾ mile	½ mile	½ mile	
Time	6 minutes	15 minutes	6 minutes	10 minutes	
Day 3	Day off				
Day 4					
Track	¾ mile	½ mile			
Time	9 minutes	10 minutes			
Day 5					
Track	¾ mile	½ mile			
Time	9 minutes	10 minutes			
Day 6	Day off				
Day 7					
Track	Mile	¾ mile			
Time	12 minutes	15 minutes			

When running on bicycle or jogging paths, the same rules of traffic apply as when driving an auto: keep to the right except when passing, and check for traffic behind you before pulling out to pass. You'll save yourself time and injuries.

PROGRAM PROCEDURES: YOUNGSTERS

SIXTH GRADE: WEEK 3

	Jog	Walk	Jog	Walk	Comments
Day 1					
Track	¾ mile	¼ mile			
Time	12 minutes	5 minutes			
Day 2					
Track	¾ mile	¼ mile			
Time	12 minutes	5 minutes			
Day 3	Day off				
Day 4					
Track	Mile	½ mile	mile	¼ mile	
Time	18 minutes	10 minutes	6 minutes	5 minutes	
Day 5					
Track	½ mile	¼ mile	½ mile	½ mile	
Time	8 minutes	5 minutes	8 minutes	10 minutes	
Day 6	Day off				
Day 7					
Track	1½ miles	½ mile	¼ mile	½ mile	
Time	24 minutes	15 minutes	3 minutes	15 minutes	

What's the best diet? Nothing beats a balanced one!

PROGRAM PROCEDURES: YOUNGSTERS

SIXTH GRADE: WEEK 4

	Jog	Walk	Jog	Walk	Comments
Day 1					
Track	¾ mile	¼ mile			
Time	12 minutes	5 minutes			
Day 2					
Track	¾ mile	¼ mile			
Time	12 minutes	5 minutes			
Day 3	Day off				
Day 4					
Track	Mile	½ mile	½ mile	¼ mile	
Time	18 minutes	10 minutes	6 minutes	5 minutes	
Day 5					
Track	½ mile	¼ mile	½ mile	½ mile	
Time	8 minutes	5 minutes	8 minutes	10 minutes	
Day 6	Day off				
Day 7					
Track	1½ mile	½ mile	¼ mile	½ mile	
Time	24 minutes	15 minutes	3 minutes	15 minutes	

Listening to your favorite music while getting ready for a run or a race is a super way to get psyched up.

PROGRAM PROCEDURES: YOUNGSTERS

SEVENTH GRADE: WEEK 1

	Jog	Walk	Jog	Walk	Comments
Day 1					
Track*	Mile	½ mile			
Time	12 minutes	10 minutes			
Day 2					
Track	Mile	¼ mile	mile	½ mile	
Time	12 minutes	5 minutes	12 minutes	10 minutes	
Day 3	Day off				
Day 4					
Track	1½ miles	½ mile	½ mile	¼ mile	
Time	18 minutes	10 minutes	6 minutes	5 minutes	
Day 5					
Track	Mile	¼ mile	mile	½ mile	
Time	12 minutes	5 minutes	12 minutes	10 minutes	
Day 6					
Track	2 miles	¾ mile	¼ mile	¼ mile	
Time	24 minutes	15 minutes	3 minutes	5 minutes	
Day 7					
Track	1½ miles	½ mile	½ mile	¼ mile	
Time	18 minutes	10 minutes	6 minutes	5 minutes	

*Use running track or measured distance. On days off, practice other sports.

Running with friends makes a workout more fun, but always be careful to run with people of the same ability as your own. Also, run at least some hard workouts alone so you won't have to depend on your group to pull you through a tough race.

PROGRAM PROCEDURES: YOUNGSTERS

SEVENTH GRADE: WEEK 2

	Jog	Walk	Jog	Walk	Comments
Day 1					
Track	Mile	½ mile			
Time	12 minutes	10 minutes			
Day 2					
Track	Mile	¼ mile	mile	½ mile	
Time	12 minutes	5 minutes	12 minutes	10 minutes	
Day 3	Day off				
Day 4					
Track	1½ miles	½ mile	½ mile	¼ mile	
Time	18 minutes	10 minutes	6 minutes	5 minutes	
Day 5					
Track	Mile	¼ mile	mile	½ mile	
Time	12 minutes	5 minutes	12 minutes	10 minutes	
Day 6					
Track	2 miles	¾ mile	¼ mile	¼ mile	
Time	24 minutes	15 minutes	3 minutes	5 minutes	
Day 7					
Track	1½ miles	½ mile	½ mile	¼ mile	
Time	18 minutes	10 minutes	6 minutes	5 minutes	

Running through lovely, crusty snow may bring out the poet in you, but it will also bring you to a doctor. It's a good way to injure your Achilles tendon.

PROGRAM PROCEDURES: YOUNGSTERS

SEVENTH GRADE: WEEK 3

	Jog	Walk	Jog	Walk	Comments
Day 1					
Track	Mile	½ mile			
Time	12 minutes	10 minutes			
Day 2					
Track	Mile	¼ mile	mile	½ mile	
Time	12 minutes	5 minutes	12 minutes	10 minutes	
Day 3	Day off				
Day 4					
Track	1½ mile	½ mile	½ mile	¼ mile	
Time	18 minutes	10 minutes	6 minutes	5 minutes	
Day 5					
Track	Mile	¼ mile	mile	½ mile	
Time	12 minutes	5 minutes	12 minutes	10 minutes	
Day 6					
Track	2 miles	¾ miles	¼ mile	¼ mile	
Time	24 minutes	15 minutes	3 minutes	5 minutes	
Day 7					
Track	1½ miles	½ mile	½ mile	¼ mile	
Time	18 minutes	10 minutes	6 minutes	5 minutes	

To Join or Not to Join

Don't hesitate to join a track club if you're at all interested. Track clubs welcome members at all levels of ability, and there's nothing like the strength of team spirit to bring out the tiger in you.

PROGRAM PROCEDURES: YOUNGSTERS

SEVENTH GRADE: WEEK 4

	Jog	Walk	Jog	Walk	Comments
Day 1					
Track	Mile	½ mile			
Time	12 minutes	10 minutes			
Day 2					
Track	Mile	¼ mile	mile	½ mile	
Time	12 minutes	5 minutes	12 minutes	10 minutes	
Day 3	Day off				
Day 4					
Track	1½ miles	½ mile	½ mile	¼ mile	
Time	18 minutes	10 minutes	6 minutes	5 minutes	
Day 5					
Track	Mile	¼ mile	mile	½ mile	
Time	12 minutes	5 minutes	12 minutes	10 minutes	
Day 6					
Track	2 miles	¾ mile	¼ mile	¼ mile	
Time	24 minutes	15 minutes	3 minutes	5 minutes	
Day 7					
Track	2 miles	½ mile			
Time	24 minutes	10 minutes			

The time to use "goo" on your shoes is before the first time you run in them. Put the liquid cement on areas you know from experience will wear down from your personal gait. It's much easier to keep a shoe from wearing down than it is to build a worn shoe back up.

PROGRAM PROCEDURES: YOUNGSTERS

EIGHTH GRADE: WEEK 1

	Jog	Walk	Jog	Walk	Comments
Day 1					
Track*	2 miles	½ mile	mile	¼ mile	
Time	24 minutes	10 minutes	12 minutes	5 minutes	
Day 2					
Track	2½ miles	½ mile			
Time	30 minutes	10 minutes			
Day 3					
Track	2 miles	½ mile	mile	¼ mile	
Time	24 minutes	10 minutes	12 minutes	5 minutes	
Day 4	Day off				
Day 5					
Track	2½ miles	½ mile			
Time	20 minutes	10 minutes			
Day 6					
Track	2 miles	mile			
Time	24 minutes	20 minutes			
Day 7					
Track	3 miles	½ mile			
Time	37 minutes	10 minutes			

*Use running track or measured distance.

A running shoe may look fine but be almost totally useless. Studies in the late 1970s and early 1980s show that many shoes lose their shock-absorbing characteristics—particularly under the forefoot—in 500 miles or less. Don't resole—replace.

PROGRAM PROCEDURES: YOUNGSTERS

EIGHTH GRADE: WEEK 2

Day	Workout	Conditions	Comments
1	3 miles		
2	2¾ miles		
3	3 miles		
4	Day off		
5	2½ miles		
6	3 miles		
7	3¼ miles		

Daily avg.:

Mileage for week:

_____

_____

_____

_____

Check out your new shoes thoroughly before leaving the store with them. Unfortunately, some companies have terrible quality control (ask your friends; most people know which companies these are). Make certain your new shoes are stable by placing them on a level table, putting your head level with the table, and looking at the shoes from the back. If both shoes don't stand up perfectly straight, buy another pair that does.

PROGRAM PROCEDURES: YOUNGSTERS

EIGHTH GRADE: WEEK 3

Day	Workout	Conditions	Comments
1	3 miles		
2	3 miles		
3	4 miles		
4	Day off		
5	3 miles		
6	3 miles		
7	4 miles		

Daily avg.:

Mileage for week:

Running on grass at night is one of the best possible ways to get injured by stepping in or tripping over something you didn't see. Not a good idea.

PROGRAM PROCEDURES: YOUNGSTERS

EIGHTH GRADE: WEEK 4

Day	Workout	Conditions	Comments
1	3 miles		
2	4 miles		
3	3 miles		
4	Day off		
5	4 miles		
6	2 miles		
7	3 miles		

Daily avg.:

Mileage for week:

_____

_____

_____

_____

Take note of the wind (direction and velocity) and humidity (relative percentage) before going on your run. These data can change drastically in less than an hour, and strongly determine how you should dress, and often even how you should run. Major cities offer weather forecasts over the telephone that provide such "surface information," as the meteorologists call it.

PROGRAM PROCEDURES: YOUNGSTERS

EIGHTH GRADE: WEEK 5

Day	Workout	Conditions	Comments
1	4 miles		
2	3 miles		
3	2 miles		
4	Day off		
5	3 miles		
6	3 miles		
7	5 miles		

Daily avg.:

Mileage for week:

11

WALKING

This chapter gives a training schedule for athletes who want to get their aerobic exercise by walking. It may also be used by runners with injuries that prevent them from running and who want to lose as little fitness as possible while injured. (The final 2 weeks of the program would probably be the most useful to the injured runner, particularly if he or she is a competitive racer.) The schedule comprises only 8 weeks of daily instruction, but you can use it for walking for years and years. Simply stop at the weekly schedule you find sufficiently demanding, then keep repeating it. Find different, interesting routes for your walking to help you maintain your enthusiasm. If you find yourself tired, walk the schedule provided for the week previous to your normal one. (For example, if you choose Week 5 as the level you want to maintain, and become tired, walk the schedule for Week 4 instead.)

The workout instructions are given in terms of minutes of walking instead of in miles to cover. In this regard, they are different from other schedules in this book. Please don't try to walk for 20 miles your first day! We want you to walk for 20 minutes. We have used this approach because how long you exercise is more important than how much ground you cover. Moreover, you will find yourself walking faster to keep your pulse in your aerobic zone as you get fitter. By phrasing the training schedules in terms of time rather than distance, we've kept them useful to you for your whole career as a walker.

SHOES FOR WALKING

Running shoes are best for walking as an exercise because they provide the kind of cushioning and heel support demanded by such concentrated, repetitive motion. Running shoes also give you better traction than your wing-tips or pumps. Some athletic-gear companies were planning to produce shoes intended especially for aerobic walking at the time we wrote this. They may by now be on the market. Ask about them at a reputable sporting goods store.

When selecting your shoes, stay away from those with the heels much higher than the front part of the shoe, because they lead to muscle and tendon injury in the back of the leg. Also beware of thickly cushioned shoes. Walkers don't need lots of cushioning. Walkers strike the ground with, at most, twice their body weight, while runners can hit the ground with up to 8 times their body weight. A thickly cushioned shoe tends to wobble around on the ground at walking speed. Furthermore, the price of a running shoe is usually directly proportionate to the cushioning it offers. Get yourself a pair of shoes intended for road racing (not track spikes!), and you should be all set.

Important note: Running shoes are not good at all for just walking around, even though we all wear them for that, too. A running shoe is designed only for rapid forward motion. They are not meant for ambling forward motion, or for any sort of lateral motion. It's very common to twist your ankle when walking around town in running shoes. You're much better off using a good court shoe—tennis, basketball, racquetball, aerobics—for such purposes. These shoes are adequately cushioned and also intended for backward and lateral motion.

TIPS FOR WALKERS

Keep at it for at least 20 minutes per workout. Gradually lengthen the time you walk. It's how long you elevate your pulse, more than how far you walk, that builds up your health.

Use your arms as well as your legs. Use your whole body when you walk. Learn to coordinate your arms and legs. Bend your arms at right angles at the elbows and swing them rhythmically. Most experts believe that it is your arm speed that determines your leg speed, not vice versa. Your arms and legs will move at exactly the same speed. If they don't, you will fall over yourself. This is a law of both physics and biomechanics. Putting your entire body into your walk not only gives you better balance and thrust, it helps tone your upper as well as lower body, resulting in even greater health.

Make sure you use both legs at all times. We're not kidding. In walking, the athlete pulls himself or herself along with the extended leg while simultaneously pushing himself or herself forward with the trailing leg. In running, all propulsion comes form one leg at a time. This is why walking develops the shin muscles and running does not.

Walking for health is not a mild stroll. This is no sissy sport. You should be doing 20-minute miles, or better. (However, you should never be going at it so hard that you cannot simultaneously carry on a normal conversation. This is a basic rule of all aerobic exercise. It's called the "talk test." If you can't talk normally, you're overdoing it, tearing yourself down instead of building yourself up.) A 20-minute mile is a speed of only 3 miles an hour. It's probably not faster than you ordinarily walk, but it may take some concentration to keep it up for a mile or more. As your fitness improves, you'll be doing 15-minute miles, 12-minute miles, and even 10-minute miles comfortably.

Walking is an excellent sport that's received less attention than it deserves because of the recent glamor surrounding running. We feel that more and more people will start to take up walking for fun and fitness. Unlike runners, walkers almost never suffer injury. Edward P. Weston, a celebrated American race-walker of the late 1800s, said that his workouts felt "like a soothing massage." Walking confers aerobic benefits while also allowing the athlete to pay some attention to enjoying his or her surroundings. You can't ask more from a sport than that.

NOTES

Exercise Pick-ups: Workouts marked with a [+] are designed to elevate your pulse rate a bit and add zest to your training. They entail walking a bit faster than your normal pace for a few minutes. They are intended strictly for fun. If you don't find them fun, then please don't do them. The symbols in the training chart are explained below.

[+]Walk at your normal pace for the first 15 minutes of your workout, then walk a bit more briskly for 4 minutes. Then finish the walk at your normal pace.

[++]Walk at your normal pace for the first 15 minutes, then walk more briskly for 4 minutes; resume your normal pace for 11 minutes, then walk briskly for 2 minutes. Finish at your normal pace.

[+++]Walk at your normal pace for the first 15 minutes, then walk more briskly for 5 minutes. Resume your normal pace for the next 5 minutes, then walk briskly again for 2 minutes. Finish at your normal pace.

[++++]Walk at your normal pace for the first 15 minutes, then walk briskly for 5 minutes. Resume normal pace for the next 5 minutes, then walk briskly for 2 minutes. Resume normal pace for the next 8 minutes, then walk briskly for 2 minutes. Resume normal pace for the next 8 minutes, then walk briskly for 3 minutes. Walk at normal pace for the next 7 minutes, then walk briskly for 2 minutes. Resume normal pace for the next 8 minutes, walk briskly for 2 minutes, and finish at your normal pace.

PROGRAM PROCEDURES: WALKING

WEEK 1

Day	Workout	Conditions	Comments
1	20 minutes		
2	23 minutes		
3	25 minutes		
4	23 minutes⁺		
5	25 minutes		
6	28 minutes		
7	25 minutes		

Daily avg.:

PROGRAM PROCEDURES: WALKING

WEEK 2

Day	Workout	Conditions	Comments
1	off		
2	28 minutes		
3	30 minutes		
4	28 minutes[+]		
5	32 minutes		
6	35 minutes		
7			

Daily avg.:

_____

_____

_____

_____

PROGRAM PROCEDURES: WALKING

WEEK 3

Day	Workout	Conditions	Comments
1	35 minutes		
2	38 minutes		
3	30 minutes$^+$		
4	40 minutes		
5	45 minutes		
6			
7			

Daily avg.:

PROGRAM PROCEDURES: WALKING

WEEK 4

Day	Workout	Conditions	Comments
1	40 minutes		
2	45 minutes		
3	35 minutes^{++}		
4	48 minutes		
5	55 minutes		
6			
7			

Daily avg.:

PROGRAM PROCEDURES: WALKING

WEEK 5

Day	Workout	Conditions	Comments
1	50 minutes		
2	55 minutes		
3	40 minutes[++]		
4	60 minutes		
5	65 minutes		
6			
7			

Daily avg.:

PROGRAM PROCEDURES: WALKING

WEEK 6

Day	Workout	Conditions	Comments
1	55 minutes		
2	60 minutes		
3	40 minutes^{++}		
4	65 minutes		
5	70 minutes		
6			
7			

Daily avg.:

PROGRAM PROCEDURES: WALKING

WEEK 7

Day	Workout	Conditions	Comments
1	60 minutes		
2	65 minutes		
3	40 minutes^{+++}		
4	70 minutes		
5	75 minutes^{++++}		
6			
7			

Daily avg.:

PROGRAM PROCEDURES: WALKING

WEEK 8

Day	Workout	Conditions	Comments
1	60 minutes		
2	70 minutes		
3	40 minutes[+++]		
4	75 minutes		
5	80 minutes[++++]		
6			
7			

Daily avg.:

12

STAGE 1: WALK, JOG, RUN (4-week program)

WALK-JOG PROGRAM

This program of progressive exercise consists of walking and jogging at a slow, moderate, or an up-tempo pace according to your own level of physical conditioning, desire, and ability. Achieving this base level will take many people from four to ten weeks of regular training. The successful jogger-to-runner is one who is able to maintain a regular program after at least four weeks without excess fatigue or injury.

How do you begin? First, find a nice, slow, and comfortable pace, settle into it, and relax. At this point, you become content. There is no need to go further. Good things are now happening to the body. Try to have one or more friends of the same age and the same physical condition join you. When you have company you enjoy the activity more. You can also compare notes, motivate one another, and have something to talk about. When you "get into running" there is a whole society out there ready to converse with you! Just remember that any good program requires time.

Consistency is the key. The beginner must become aware that consistent running, no matter how slow the pace or how short the distance, is the easiest and fastest path to fitness. A little running is better than no running at all. Rationalizations for skipping a few workouts are very easy to find. Don't give in to them.

Initially, you should set a daily exercise goal not in terms of minutes run or distance completed, but in the seemingly easy step of just making the initial commitment by wanting to get some exercise, getting dressed to run, and leaving the house. If a beginner can just get out the door on a consistent basis, then fitness is virtually a certainty.

Consistent running does not mean that you must work out every day, regardless of the circumstances. Though four or five days running per week are necessary for a training effect, one day off every one or two weeks is reasonable and necessary for most people. Family emergencies, extreme weather conditions, illness, and injury must not be overlooked. A day off from running sometimes pro-

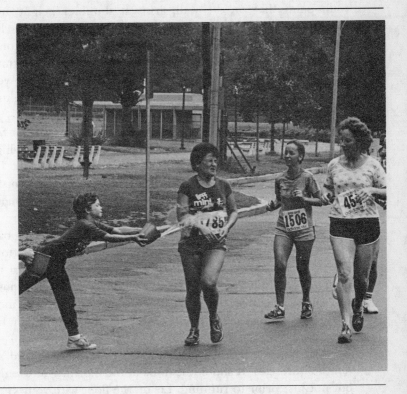

Run well and make a splash with your friends! It's essential to keep cool during even the shorter-distance events, such as this 5-mile road race. If you're doused during hard exertion, however, make certain the water lands either on your midriff (as here) or on your head. Wet feet become blistered, and a suddenly wet chest can lead to cardiac arrest! (Photograph courtesy of George J. Marcelonis)

vides a refreshing mental and physical pause in the normal daily routine that will actually serve to enhance running.

Proper Stretching Exercises

1. *Toe touching:* Cross legs right over left. Bend from the waist to the ankle, hands touching the peat three times. Then do left over right.
2. *Wall push-up:* This exercise is good for the calf muscles. Stand flat-footed about three feet from the wall. Lean forward toward wall, palms flat on the wall, arms at shoulder height, until muscles feel tightened. Keeping the knees locked, the legs straight, and the feet flat, hold the position for two seconds, gradually increase to five seconds. Relax. Repeat three times.
3. *Adductor stretch:* Stand straight with feet wide and let your hands gently slide down your leg toward your right ankle until you feel the stretch. Do five times with each leg.
4. *Hurdler's stretch:* While standing, place the heel of right foot on a bench or some other object at least eighteen inches high. Keep your knee straight and point your toe straight up. The left leg remains straight and locked at the knee with foot flat on floor. Gently reach down your right leg with both hands and try to touch your toes. Do five times with each leg.
5. *Quad or thigh stretch:* Stand up straight and bend one leg back at the knee so that your heel is pressing against your buttock. Then, keeping your trunk straight and your heel against the buttock, get your thighs as parallel with one another as possible. Grab the ankle, but don't force to the buttock. The more advanced athlete will find this exercise easier. Hold for five seconds. Do five times with each leg.
6. *Bent-leg sit-up:* Here's a good one to develop back and abdominal muscles. It should be done in the morning or evening but not just prior to running. Lie on the floor with your knees bent and your feet close to your buttocks. Come to a sitting position. Lie back. Repeat until you can't do any more or up to twenty times.

To lessen the risk of injury, runners should work daily for flexibility. Certainly, no one should run without warming up first. Some runners zip through their stretching routine in five or ten minutes; others may take a half-hour. You are the best judge of how much warm-up time your body needs. A loose, stretched muscle feels different from a tight, inflexible one. Focus your attention on your muscles when you are warming up and learn to identify that warm, tingly, stretched-out feeling. Most running injuries are due to tight inflexible muscles, so stretching and proper warm-ups are important.

The new runner should try the following warm-up. First do stretching exercises, then a slow ten-minute jog, then proceed to a normal speed for the amount of time that you feel comfortable. A more experienced runner or one who is about to roll can follow a different procedure. First, do your stretching and then twelve minutes of slow jog, followed by two pick-ups (from jogging pace to three-quarter pace to race pace) for fifty to seventy-five yards. This should be sufficient warm-up for most runners.

A proper warm-up is scientifically beneficial because it raises your maximum oxygen capacity level, lowers lactic acid, and produces a higher heart rate and higher muscle temperature. In this condition, the body is ready for a quick surge at race start.

Warm-up

Learning to endure pain isn't nearly as much fun as learning to prevent injury altogether. That's why warm-up exercises are so important. Tendons are more easily torn and injured if muscles are tight. If the muscles are stretched and flexible, tendons don't have to carry so much of the strain and the chance of tendonitis is greatly reduced.

You should concentrate on loosening these primary muscle groups: the calf muscles (women's tend to be especially tight), the hamstrings (the posterior thigh muscles), and the quadriceps (the anterior thigh muscle).

Frequently, overuse injuries show up as tendonitis, which is an inflammation of the tendon or the sheath (sleeve) that surrounds it. Tendons attach muscle to bone. Though medical science isn't certain about what causes tendonitis, it is probably due to microscopic tears in the tendon, which cause pain and swelling. Tendons have a poor blood supply. They take a long time to heal and are easily reinjured. It may take a runner with tendonitis a year or more to heal completely. Take heed! Remember that fact!

Most running injuries are caused by overuse. Tendons tear, muscles rip, joints wear out because runners try to do too much, too soon, and for too long. Running is a highly individualistic sport, and what is too much for one person may not be quite enough for another. That's why the first step in running is the warm-up.

Warm-down

The value of a five-minute cool-down after exercising is that it makes the rest of your day much more enjoyable and helps you avoid the aches, pains, and cramps that otherwise might wake you up in the middle of the night and make you miserable.

A cool-down allows your body to flush away the toxins that build up when you exercise. As you burn energy, fuel in the form of glucose (sugar) in the muscles is consumed. The end product of glucose metabolism is lactic acid. If you suddenly stop running and sit down, blood will pool in your legs and the lactic acid will not be cleared. It's the lactic acid that is responsible for most of the muscle aches you get the day after exercise. To avoid this problem, jog slowly, walk around, and stretch for five minutes or so after you run. Some people eliminate the stretching and still feel fine. You decide what makes your body feel best.

Getting back in groove after a few years of not running may require starting with this program: try to walk three miles in forty-five minutes; when you have reached that stage, you are ready to begin a jogging program.

There is a direct relationship between oxygen uptake and the energy demands that are placed on the body. The less energy being expended, the lower the level of oxygen consumption. As a person begins to exercise at a relatively steady level, as in jogging, oxygen consumption goes through a transition state that lasts from three to six minutes. It then levels off and maintains this new level as long as the same intensity of exercise continues. If the intensity of the exercise changes, the oxygen uptake level will also change. There is a linear relationship between exercise intensity and the steady level of oxygen consumption. Eventually you can achieve a level of exercise in which you cannot increase oxygen intake any more, and exhaustion follows. Normally, however, the cells receive the oxygen that they need at any level of submaximal exercise.

PROGRAM PROCEDURES: WALK, JOG, RUN

STAGE 1: WEEK 1

	Jog	Walk	Jog	Walk	Comments
Day 1					
Track*	½ mile	¾ mile	½ mile	½ mile	
Time	6 minutes	15 minutes	6 minutes	10 minutes	
Day 2					
Track	½ mile	¾ mile	½ mile	½ mile	
Time	6 minutes	15 minutes	6 minutes	10 minutes	
Day 3					
Track	¾ mile	½ mile	½ mile	½ mile	
Time	9 minutes	10 minutes	6 minutes	10 minutes	
Day 4					
Track	¾ mile	½ mile	¾ mile	½ mile	
Time	9 minutes	10 minutes	9 minutes	10 minutes	
Day 5					
Track	Mile	¾ mile	½ mile	½ mile	
Time	12 minutes	15 minutes	6 minutes	10 minutes	
Day 6					
Track	Mile	½ mile	Mile	½ mile	
Time	12 minutes	6 minutes	12 minutes	6 minutes	
Day 7	Day off				

*Use running track or measured distance.

I Don't Have Time Today

The time you spend running could be utilized by watching a game or a soap opera on TV. But physically and mentally, you will be the loser. So dress quickly and run for the door before you change your mind.

You are sore, it's been a long time. The price for conditioning will be discomfort for the following ten days. But then!

PROGRAM PROCEDURES: WALK, JOG, RUN

STAGE 1: WEEK 2

	Jog	Walk	Jog	Walk	Comments
Day 1					
Track	Mile	¼ mile	mile	½ mile	
Time	12 minutes	5 minutes	12 minutes	10 minutes	
Day 2					
Track	Mile	¼ mile	mile	½ mile	
Time	12 minutes	5 minutes	12 minutes	10 minutes	
Day 3					
Track	1½ miles	½ mile	½ mile	¼ mile	
Time	18 minutes	10 minutes	6 minutes	5 minutes	
Day 4					
Track	Mile	¼ mile	mile	½ mile	
Time	12 minutes	5 minutes	12 minutes	10 minutes	
Day 5					
Track	2 miles	¾ mile	¼ mile	¼ mile	
Time	24 minutes	15 minutes	3 minutes	5 minutes	
Day 6					
Track	1½ miles	½ mile	½ mile	¼ mile	
Time	18 minutes	10 minutes	6 minutes	5 minutes	
Day 7	Day off				

It's **Hot** *Today*

Heat is the number-one enemy of long-distance runners. It dehydrates the body. But if you drink a large glass of water one-half hour before you run or stop at a gas station, drinking fountain, fire station, or police station for a drink en route, you will be all right. Another drink will feel great when you arrive home.

PROGRAM PROCEDURES: WALK, JOG, RUN

STAGE 1: WEEK 3

	Jog	Walk	Jog	Walk	Comments
Day 1					
Track	2 miles	¾ mile			
Time	24 minutes	15 minutes			
Day 2					
Track	2 miles	½ mile	½ mile	¼ mile	
Time	24 minutes	10 minutes	6 minutes	5 minutes	
Day 3					
Track	2 miles	¾ mile	¼ mile	¼ mile	
Time	24 minutes	15 minutes	3 minutes	5 minutes	
Day 4					
Track	2¼ miles	½ mile			
Time	27 minutes	10 minutes			
Day 5					
Track	2 miles	½ mile			
Time	24 minutes	10 minutes			
Day 6					
Track	2½ miles	½ mile			
Time	30 minutes	10 minutes			

Day 7   Optional day off

I Might Be Injured *If I Run That Far!*

Sure, you might be run over by a car. A dog might bite you. You might sprain your ankle. You might also get lost on a new route.

The primary objective of running is fitness. Being physically fit means being in condition, *that is, being capable of sustaining high-level total body efforts for a period of time. To allow such effort, the heart and cardiovascular system must be in top condition in order to transport the necessary oxygen from the lungs to the active muscles.*

PROGRAM PROCEDURES: WALK, JOG, RUN

STAGE 1: WEEK 4

	Jog	Walk	Jog	Walk	Comments
Day 1					
Track	2 miles	½ mile	mile	¼ mile	
Time	24 minutes	10 minutes	12 minutes	5 minutes	
Day 2					
Track	2½ miles	½ mile			
Time	30 minutes	10 minutes			
Day 3					
Track	2 miles	½ mile	mile	¼ mile	
Time	24 minutes	10 minutes	12 minutes	5 minutes	
Day 4					
Track	2½ miles	½ mile			
Time	20 minutes	10 minutes			
Day 5					
Track	2 miles	mile			
Time	24 minutes	20 minutes			
Final track					
Track	3 miles	½ mile			
Time	37 minutes	10 minutes			

Graduate to runner

It's Raining

Afraid you'll get wet and catch cold or maybe pneumonia? Wrong! You won't if you take a shower as soon as you have finished running. Besides, the rain is great for your hair!

P.S. Colds and pneumonia are caused by viruses.

13

STAGE 2F: RUNNING FOR BASIC FITNESS (13-week program)

If you want to run for fun, fitness, and health; if you want to integrate running into a more comprehensive exercise program; or if you want to use running as a supplementary exercise to attain greater excellence in another sport—this is the program for you.

The schedule is designed for people with limited time available for running. You'll notice that at no time do you run more than 5 days in a week's training, and usually only 4 days a week, whereas the schedules intended for competitive racers require them to run 6 or 7 days a week. It is certainly safe to run more often than 4 or 5 times a week. We simply figured that athletes who are using running as part of a larger fitness program would be working out at other athletics—or perhaps even at their careers—the rest of the week.

It is not necessary to run 4 or 5 days in a row, although the workout days follow one after the other in the schedule's charts. We've designed these schedules to provide the flexibility that *your* work and leisure schedule requires. It's okay to run a day, take two days off, then run 3 more days, then another day off. Just get in your 4 or 5 workouts each 7-day period.

It *is* necessary to run the workouts sequentially, that is, to run only the distance scheduled for the ordinal running day of that week. To use Week 1 as an example, suppose you ran 3 miles on Monday, then did other things Tuesday and Wednesday. Come Thursday, you might feel sufficiently strong to be tempted to run more than the 2 miles scheduled for running day number 2. Don't. Run the 2 miles—so you'll be well enough rested to run the 3 miles, then the 4 miles, later in the week.

You'll notice a quirk in the mileage progression from Week 9 to Week 10. Up until that point, the mileage has been building steadily. From Week 9 to Week 10, the week's total mileage *drops* by 6 miles. Over the remaining weeks of the schedule, the mileage builds up again until returning to 26 miles a week. We took this approach as a means of providing maximal training benefits for the athlete with very limited time. You'll notice that something else drops off between Week 9 and Week 10—the number of days per week that you run. It drops from 5 days to 4 days per week. This means you're running a higher daily average mileage in the last 4 weeks of the schedule. This frees up more days for you to do other things.

However, *do not* try to jump directly from Week 9 to Week 13 of the schedule. The weekly mileage is the same in both weeks, but Week 13 requires a significantly higher fitness level than does Week 9. That is why we offer a 3-week progression between the two of them. We mention this because, as with any other schedule in this book, you can choose your own cut-off point with this program. Let's say you're happy running 26 miles on a 5-day-a-week schedule, but you've got a busy week coming up, and you don't want to degenerate into quivering flab because you can run only 4 days during it. Run the schedule for Week 10 in that case, not for Week 13. Your mileage will drop, but your fitness will not. (See also Chapter 18 for more discussion on maintaining fitness.)

This program actually subdivides into three different, sequentially progressive, programs that take your time for running into account. Weeks 1 through 4 constitute the first subprogram. It requires you to devote only 4 days a week to running. Weeks 5 through 9 are for two different sorts of personal schedule: The first is that of the runner who wants to run 5 days a week, but does not want to run the kind of mileage scheduled in Chapter 16, Running for Advanced Fitness. The second is that of the runner who wants the benefits of mileage higher than offered by the end of Week 4, but who normally has only 4 days a week for running. If this second type of runner will give us only 5 days a week for 5 weeks, he or she can then run 4 days a week for the rest of his or her athletic life, but have the benefits of the higher mileage by moving on to Weeks 10 through 13.

PROGRAM PROCEDURES: BASIC FITNESS

STAGE 2F: WEEK 1

Day	Workout	Conditions	Comments
1	3 miles		
2	2 miles		
3	3 miles		
4	4 miles		
5			
6			
7			

Daily avg.: _____

Mileage for week: _____

_____

_____

_____

_____

PROGRAM PROCEDURES: BASIC FITNESS

STAGE 2F: WEEK 2

Day	Workout	Conditions	Comments
1	3 miles		
2	3 miles		
3	2 miles		
4	5 miles		
5			
6			
7			

Daily avg.:

Mileage for week:

PROGRAM PROCEDURES: BASIC FITNESS

STAGE 2F: WEEK 3

Day	Workout	Conditions	Comments
1	3 miles		
2	3 miles		
3	3 miles		
4	5 miles		
5			
6			
7			

Daily avg.:

Mileage for week:

PROGRAM PROCEDURES: BASIC FITNESS

STAGE 2F: WEEK 4

Day	Workout	Conditions	Comments
1	3 miles		
2	3 miles		
3	3 miles		
4	6 miles		
5			
6			
7			

Daily avg.:

Mileage for week:

PROGRAM PROCEDURES: BASIC FITNESS

STAGE 2F: WEEK 5

Day	Workout	Conditions	Comments
1	2 miles		
2	3 miles		
3	3 miles		
4	2 miles		
5	6 miles		
6			
7			

Daily avg.:

Mileage for week:

PROGRAM PROCEDURES: BASIC FITNESS

STAGE 2F: WEEK 6

Day	Workout	Conditions	Comments
1	3 miles		
2	4 miles		
3	3 miles		
4	2 miles		
5	6 miles		
6			
7			

Daily avg.:

Mileage for week:

PROGRAM PROCEDURES: BASIC FITNESS

STAGE 2F: WEEK 7

Day	Workout	Conditions	Comments
1	3 miles		
2	4 miles		
3	3 miles		
4	3 miles		
5	7 miles		
6			
7			

Daily avg.:

Mileage for week:

PROGRAM PROCEDURES: BASIC FITNESS

STAGE 2F: WEEK 8

Day	Workout	Conditions	Comments
1	3 miles		
2	5 miles		
3	3 miles		
4	3 miles		
5	8 miles		
6			
7			

Daily avg.:

Mileage for week:

PROGRAM PROCEDURES: BASIC FITNESS

STAGE 2F: WEEK 9

Day	Workout	Conditions	Comments
1	3 miles		
2	6 miles		
3	3 miles		
4	4 miles		
5	10 miles		
6			
7			

Daily avg.:

Mileage for week:

PROGRAM PROCEDURES: BASIC FITNESS

STAGE 2F: WEEK 10

Day	Workout	Conditions	Comments
1	4 miles		
2	5 miles		
3	4 miles		
4	7 miles		
5			
6			
7			

Daily avg.:

Mileage for week:

PROGRAM PROCEDURES: BASIC FITNESS

STAGE 2F: WEEK 11

Day	Workout	Conditions	Comments
1	4 miles		
2	5 miles		
3	4 miles		
4	8 miles		
5			
6			
7			

Daily avg.:

Mileage for week:

PROGRAM PROCEDURES: BASIC FITNESS

STAGE 2F: WEEK 12

Day	Workout	Conditions	Comments
1	4 miles		
2	7 miles		
3	5 miles		
4	9 miles		
5			
6			
7			

Daily avg.:

Mileage for week:

PROGRAM PROCEDURES: BASIC FITNESS

STAGE 2F: WEEK 13

Day	Workout	Conditions	Comments
1	4 miles		
2	7 miles		
3	5 miles		
4	10 miles		
5			
6			
7			

Daily avg.:

Mileage for week:

14

STAGE 2R: FUN RUNS (4-week program)

FUN RUN CONCEPT

One of the first things that a new runner wants to do is to complete a run of a particular distance. A fun run is just that. It is a run of a particular distance with no time limits, so the new runner doesn't face competition—just companionship! It allows you to set a goal and to complete it at your own rate of speed. That's why it is fun. It's good for setting and meeting short-term goals. Fun runs are publicized by the TAC and/or local running clubs. They're very informal, a good way to meet people, some of whom may run at your own level, and a source of information.

AEROBIC TRAINING: WHAT DOES IT DO?

The greatest benefit of aerobic work is the increase in capillarization that accompanies endurance training. It brings blood flow closer to the individual muscle fibers, thus promoting more efficient exchange of nutrients between the blood and the working muscle. From this effect, it follows that capillarization will increase in those muscles that are actually exercised, while those that are not show little or no change.

However, quite possibly one of the major shortcomings of distance running training has been the overemphasis on pure aerobic work.

Not that aerobic performance (maximum oxygen uptake) is not a crucial factor in endurance performance. Obviously, it is; but many athletes quite possibly concentrate on this aspect of training instead of spending their time more profitably on other forms of training. We will try the other training techniques as we move toward longer distance and you gain a base of strength.

WOMEN ON THE RUN

More and more women are trying distance running and finding themselves remarkably well-suited for it both physically and mentally. A woman in top condition carries nearly 20 percent of her body weight in fat, and approximately 35 percent in muscle. A male in top condition will be less than 10 percent fat, and 40 percent muscle. The differences translate into better strength and speed for males but better endurance for women. In running long distances, the body depletes its glycogen, the fuel that drives a runner. When distance runners "hit the wall"—the sudden weakness that often hits at about the eighteen-mile mark—they have run out of glycogen. Stored fat is then burned and the extra fat carried by women gives them something of an advantage. There is a 7-minute difference in men's and women's world bests in the marathon. Women are running faster each year in long-distance events. It's noted that a regular running program can decidedly improve a woman runner's strength by as much as 50 percent without a corresponding increase in size of muscles in legs, arms, and chest. Rather, good regular running accomplishes a "repackaging" of muscles and fat and helps reducing.

There is no earthly reason for a female runner to train one iota differently from a male runner. A woman's joint-connective fibers are somewhat looser than a man's. Perhaps this may mean a woman might want to avoid running on hard surfaces frequently—but that's also a wise rule for a male. When one digests all the special "women's running" articles and magazines that have inundated the market in the past decade, one comes to the not-astonishing conclusion there *is* no difference between the male and female runner other than the difference of muscle mass and weight distribution. Women do not even need a diet different from men, popular superstition notwithstanding.

In practical training terms, the difference in muscle mass results in

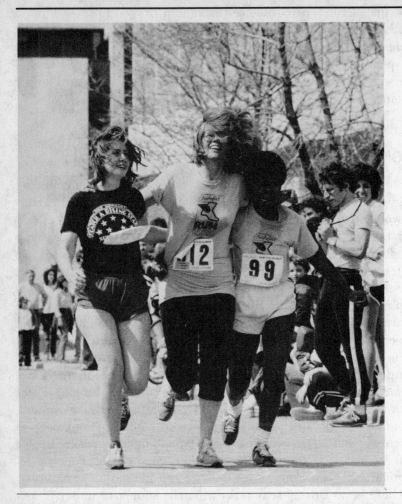

You're extra special to yourself and your friends when you finish your
first fun run. (Photograph by Bill Boyle)

one distinction between men and women training as competitive runners. A man can simply run faster than a woman (a sterling point to keep in mind if you are accosted by even a flabby-looking man during your workout—sad but true, the guy can probably outsprint you, and rapists are not interested in running a "sporting" long-distance pursuit). As a consequence, it is easier for a man to put in high mileage than it is for a woman, unless the woman is a profes-sional runner and is paid to run her workouts. Top-notch women runners seldom put in more than 80 miles a week, while world-class men often put in 50 to 100 percent more mileage than that. Still, if Allison Roe can run 2:26 at Boston in 1981 on an average of 70 miles a week, this one distinction between men and women does not seem particularly important or debilitating to the female athlete— especially in light of the fact that Roe's runner-up was running at least twice Roe's mileage. Regardless of one's sex, quality beats quantity any day.

RELAXATION OFF THE ROAD

Life brings tensions, which can build up. Collapsing on a bed and even sleeping won't always get rid of them, so when you start waking up tired in the morning, it's time to figure out ways to relax at night.

Relaxing is theoretically as natural as breathing. It's a fact that muscles relax automatically after each contraction. Tenseness interferes with relaxation, though, so it will take some conscious effort for you to do what should come naturally. Try "thinking" relaxation. Here's the method:

> Find a quiet place, loosen tight clothes, and get comfortable. Close your eyes; let your body go totally limp; breathe deeply and evenly. Slowly make a tight fist with your right hand. Tense the muscles in the right forearm and hand until they tremble. Hold for five to seven seconds to feel the muscle contractions all the way up to your shoulder. That's tension. As you unclasp the fist, focus on feeling the muscles go limp. That's relaxation.

Use this procedure for other parts of your body. First consciously tense and then consciously relax—area by area. Begin with the forehead, then eyes, jaws, neck, shoulders, arms, chest, abdomen, thighs, legs, feet, back of head and neck, and finally the back. To tense up, try frowning, gritting your teeth, pulling against the surface you're sitting or lying on, or bending arms and legs at the joints. Practice going systematically over the whole body, and soon you'll be able to relax just by willing it.

Another relaxation procedure is to breathe slowly and fully in and out, taking special care to exhale deeply and completely. This is *not* the same as hyperventilation, which is quite dangerous unless practiced by a trained expert. The inhaled breaths are *not* deep ones; they take in no more air than a normal breath. The basis of this procedure lies in the fact that all the body's muscles relax slightly and involuntarily every time we exhale. It may take several minutes to achieve full relaxation by this process, but relaxation will inevitably come—especially if you don't get anxious about it.

You'll find that being able to relax your muscles consciously will actually help relieve your psychological tensions too. If you catch yourself tensing up during the day, check to see which muscles are tensing and relax that part. You'll discover that facial muscles are usually the guilty ones, so try to remember to laugh more. Laughter relaxes the whole body.

You'll notice a change when you become adept at relaxing. Your face and eyes will look less strained. Your walk will become lighter and more graceful, and you won't feel tired all the time.

PROGRAM PROCEDURES: FUN RUNS

STAGE 2R: WEEK 1

Day	Workout	Conditions	Comments
1	3 miles		
2	2¾ miles		
3	3 miles		
4	2½ miles		
5	3 miles		
6	3¼ miles		
7			

Daily avg.:

Mileage for week:

Pollution Is Out There Today and They're Talking about Its Effects

Pollution is out there every day. Your stronger lungs gained from running will help you ward off viral infections.

PROGRAM PROCEDURES: FUN RUNS

STAGE 2R: WEEK 2

Day	Workout	Conditions	Comments
1	3 miles		
2	3 miles		
3	4 miles		
4	3 miles		
5	3 miles		
6	5 miles		
7			

Daily avg.: _____

Mileage for week: _____

_____

_____

_____

_____

I Feel Tired Today

There is an energy shortage, but it's not in your body. Eat some cookies or fruit for energy.

   Food for thought: Remember that 70 to 80 percent of the body's heat comes from food. If you tend to chill easily, you might want to experiment with food. Perhaps eating a carbohydrate snack before you run, with adequate time to digest, or eating some after you return will prevent chilling.

PROGRAM PROCEDURES: FUN RUNS

STAGE 2R: WEEK 3

Day	Workout	Conditions	Comments
1	3 miles		
2	4 miles		
3	3 miles		
4	5 miles		
5	2 miles		
6	3 miles		
7			

Daily avg.:

Mileage for week:

_____

_____

_____

_____

I Had a Headache This Morning So I'd Better Not Push Myself for the Rest of the Day

Psychologists tell us that twenty minutes of running relieves tension—a no-cost treatment.

The trunk is essentially erect during running. Excessive forward lean of the trunk places an undesirable strain on the postural muscles, creates greater force on the foot at foot strike, and hinders the forward swing of the foot and leg.

PROGRAM PROCEDURES: FUN RUNS

STAGE 2R: WEEK 4

Day	Workout	Conditions	Comments
1	5 miles		
2	3 miles		
3	5 miles		
4	4 miles		
5	3½ miles		
6	3 miles		
7			

Daily avg.:

Mileage for week:

3-mile run: write to local Athletics Congress (TAC) office for location.
Note: 1½ mile warm-up, 1½ mile warm-down before each race plus light stretching.

It's Windy Today

Running on a windy day is a great way to gain a tan or windburn without going to the ski slope.

Run into the wind to begin with, before getting too sweaty. When you run home, you will have your back to the wind so it won't go through you. Running into the wind is arduous and should be done when you are fresh, rather than on your return when you are likely to be more fatigued.

A moisturizing protective cream or suntan lotion should be applied to the face, especially to the nose, lips, and cheeks, to prevent chapping and drying. If strong winds are a factor, petroleum jelly or vegetable oil should be applied to protect against more serious complications such as frostbite.

15

STAGE 3R: TEN-KILOMETER RACE (12-week program)

PRERACE SLEEP

Everyone talks about prerace meals, but you won't go anywhere if you are tired!

Rules: Get ready for a good sleep two nights before THE BIG DAY. The following activities will help:

1. Walking several hours before bedtime is great for digestion and legs.
2. Do something routine in the hour before bed, like reading a book or watching a TV program.
3. Don't bring thoughts about the race into your bedroom.
4. If you find that you can't sleep, don't stay in bed. Get up, go sit in a chair, and read.
5. Don't sleep in a warm room or a very dry room.
6. Try to eliminate outside noise.
7. Your training should make you confident, so relax yourself.

Tips: Positive thinking plus a light snack may make you feel comfortable.

167

THE FIRST RACE

As you prepare for your first race, you need to consider several details. First, avoid wearing a new pair of shoes for the first race. Wear your new shoes several times prior to a race because they may cause blisters and, therefore, pain. Needless to say, with blisters you'll never run at your top performance level. Next, remember that clothes are important. When competing in moderate or warm temperatures, you should wear a mesh top or T-shirt and shorts. In the winter, a hat and gloves, a long-sleeved shirt or a sweat suit, and a windbreaker are usually sufficient. Do not overdress, as your body heat will keep you warm. Materials vary according to preference. Be sure the fit of your clothes doesn't restrict movement.

Think about packing your bag the night before your race. Remember to include running shoes, Vaseline (for antichafing protection), extra pins for your number, comb, and soap (so you won't be without if it is not provided at the after-the-race shower). Also take clean shorts, shirt, socks, and extra shoelaces. You might take some liquids in a thermos bottle to drink before or at the conclusion of the race. ERG or water is recommended. Race applications generally state if there are no dressing facilities at the race site. Plan accordingly. Come dressed to run.

On the morning of the race, you might find yourself making a few trips to the bathroom. Don't worry about it. It's just part of the prerace jitters. Eating breakfast is a matter of choice. Some people prefer to run a short race on an empty stomach. Others feel better when they have had something light, like pancakes.

Attempt to arrive at the meet site at least an hour before the scheduled run. Get into your running gear if you haven't already done so. Apply Vaseline to areas where your shirt, shorts, and shoes may rub. Check in and pick up your number. If at all possible, review a map of the course or drive the course to familiarize yourself with the terrain if you haven't done so previously. This awareness will assist in the completion of your first run! Jog the last half mile of the course to warm up.

Approximately one-half hour prior to the start of the race begin your warm-up. Some stretching exercises and jogging will be adequate. At the conclusion of the warm-up, check your shoelaces and double-knot them so they won't give you any problems.

When the call is given to line up, retreat to the rear of the pack of

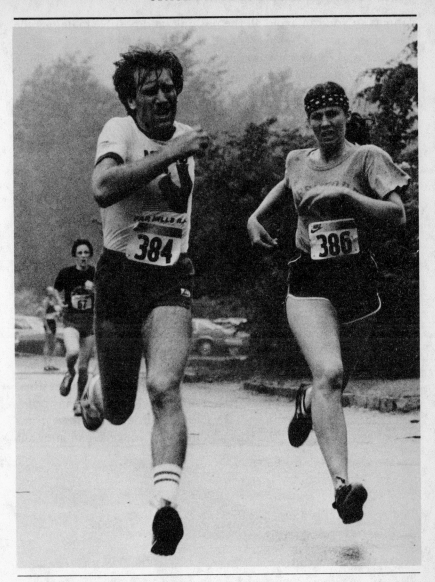

In a first race, the goal should be to finish and feel good about it, rather than to be concerned about good running form. (Photograph by Bill Boyle)

runners so you can avoid all the pushing (and possible falling) at the start of the race.

At the start of the race, don't sprint out with the rest of the field of runners. Begin with a comfortable relaxed pace—one that you have maintained throughout your conditioning program will be sufficient. You will enjoy the race a great deal more if you forget about the runners in front of you and concentrate on your own goal. You can be assured there will be others in the race who are new to racing.

If you should feel that you want to give up, don't, unless you are really hurting. We have all had the feeling at one time or another that we would like to stop, but we have finished the race. Attempt to keep your thoughts positive and omit the negative. With the approach of the finish line, a feeling of exhilaration will come over you. You have accomplished your goal, and all the problems you might have had during the race are gone. It will all have further meaning when you discuss the race at a later date.

If at all possible, stay for the awards ceremony. As you return home, you might want to review the race. Did I do what I set out to do? How about my condition? Do I need more mileage? How about another race? Upon arriving at home, consider taking a warm bath. It is not uncommon for runners to be stiff or sore the day following the race. You might want to train at a more gentle pace than usual for the next few days. Don't push yourself too hard, and any aches will soon begin to disappear. Review your first race and you are guaranteed to come to the conclusion that it wasn't so bad after all!

PROGRAM PROCEDURES: TEN-KILOMETER RACE

STAGE 3R: WEEK 1

Day	Workout	Conditions	Comments
1	4 miles		
2	6 miles		
3	4 miles		
4	6 miles		
5	4 miles		
6	8 miles		
7			

Daily avg.:

Mileage for week:

Note: On the long run, time the first half of the run and retrace the distance at a slightly faster tempo. Do not try to race distance or push yourself too hard.

Now a Runner

A jogger lifts his or her weight off the ground but does not spend as much time airborne as the runner. Beyond a certain point, usually close to a speed of nine miles per hour, you will have both feet off the ground for a longer period of time. At this point, jogging becomes running. Running means trying to reach a particular place or cover a certain distance in the shortest feasible length of time.

NOTES

Speed Pick-ups: These workouts will simulate race conditions. After you warm up, follow this procedure:

FIRST SESSION
1.   Run for 20 seconds at 95 percent effort.
2.   Rest for four minutes and forty seconds.
3.   Do this five times.

SUBSEQUENT SESSIONS
1.   Add ten seconds to the previous effort. This cuts down the rest time.
2.   Do this five times.
3.   The ideal goal would be seven repetitions of one minute with four minutes rest.
4.   The ultimate goal is eight repetitions for two minutes. This is only done by national caliber athletes.

Hill Training: Hill Training builds speed, strength, and knee lift which are needed in the latter part of races. Procedure:
1.   Find a hill 120 yards long. You must be able to run down it safely with no excess strain to knees, ankles, and hips.
2.   Warm up for thirty minutes.
3.   Place marking on hill at 50, 70, 90, and 120 yard distances.
4.   Run up and back to the 50 yard mark three times. Repeat at the 70 yard mark twice, at the 90 yard mark once, and at the 120 yard mark once.
5.   Take a twenty minute warm-down.
6.   You may become proficient enough to repeat this total procedure. If so, jog for three minutes, then repeat the workout partially or totally.

PROGRAM PROCEDURES: TEN-KILOMETER RACE

STAGE 3R: WEEK 2

Day	Workout	Conditions	Comments
1	4 miles		
2	6 miles*		
3	4 miles		
4	6 miles		
5	4 miles		
6	8 miles		
7			

Daily avg.:

Mileage for week:

*See Notes, p. 172.

Relax

Upon returning from your run, relax with your feet up at least five to six inches above the rest of your body for at least four or five minutes, sip a glass of water or juice, a cup of tea, or a liquid of your choice even if you do not feel thirsty. You are as vulnerable to dehydration in the winter as you are in the summer.

PROGRAM PROCEDURES: TEN-KILOMETER RACE

STAGE 3R: WEEK 3

Day	Workout	Conditions	Comments
1	4 miles		
2	6 miles		
3	4 miles*		
4	5 miles		
5	5 miles		
6	8 miles (race a 5- or 6-miler)		
7			

Daily avg.:

Mileage for week:

*See Notes, p. 172.

Run where there is less chance of encountering vehicles, such as in parks. I recommend running in large parking lots, such as the ones surrounding shopping malls, especially when it snows. They are usually well-lighted and plowed.

PROGRAM PROCEDURES: TEN-KILOMETER RACE

STAGE 3R: WEEK 4

Day	Workout	Conditions	Comments
1	6 miles**		
2	4 miles		
3	9 miles*		
4	6 miles		
5	4 miles		
6	9 miles*		
7			

Daily avg.:

Mileage for week:

*See Notes, p. 172.
**See Notes, p. 172.

Whatever your level of fitness, your training motto should be: "Train, don't strain." Take the "talk test" while running: if you're breathing too hard to carry on a conversation, you're going too fast.

PROGRAM PROCEDURES: TEN-KILOMETER RACE

STAGE 3R: WEEK 5

Day	Workout	Conditions	Comments
1	6 miles		
2	4 miles		
3	9 miles*		
4	6 miles		
5	4 miles		
6	9 miles*		
7			

Daily avg.:

Mileage for week:

_____

_____

_____

_____

*See Notes, p. 172.

Warm up and cool down. Start slowly, even if you're an experienced runner, for the first three or four minutes of your run. Then work up to the speed or effort you want to maintain for the entire training session. For the last three or four minutes of your run, slow down to help prevent muscle stiffness the next day.

PROGRAM PROCEDURES: TEN-KILOMETER RACE

STAGE 3R: WEEK 6

Day	Workout	Conditions	Comments
1	6 miles		
2	4 miles		
3	9 miles		
4	5 miles		
5	3 miles		
6	9 miles		
7			

Daily avg.:

Mileage for week:

After ten weeks of training, you can expect to see, among other things: a slower heart rate, increased heart stroke volume, lower blood pressure, lower cholesterol, more lipoproteins (now thought to provide protection against coronary disease), weight loss, increased work capacity, and increased lean body weight.

PROGRAM PROCEDURES: TEN-KILOMETER RACE

STAGE 3R: WEEK 7

Day	Workout	Condition	Comments
1	6 miles		
2	8 miles*		
3	6 miles		
4	8 miles		
5	6 miles		
6	10 miles*		
7			

Daily avg.:

Mileage for week:

_____

_____

_____

_____

*See Notes, p. 172.

Body Development

Do fifteen push-ups twice per day to develop arms, shoulders, and back.

Do thirty bent-knee sit-ups per day, preferably in the evening, to develop abdomen, thigh muscles, and back.

Stretching

Include stretching exercises in the warm-up.

Avoid bouncing exercises and jerky muscle contractions that exert excessive tension on muscle fibers and connective tissue.

PROGRAM PROCEDURES: TEN-KILOMETER RACE

STAGE 3R: WEEK 8

Day	Workout	Conditions	Comments
1	6 miles		
2	8 miles		
3	6 miles		
4	8 miles		
5	6 miles		
6	10 miles**		
7			

Daily avg.:

Mileage for week:

_____

_____

_____

_____

**See Notes, p. 172.

Running on Roads

Avoid running too much in one direction on a slanted road. Your body compensates in an effort to hold you erect, and this effort often leads to hip, ankle, and foot problems. If all your roads are rounded, try to run an equal amount on opposite slants.

PROGRAM PROCEDURES: TEN-KILOMETER RACE

STAGE 3R: WEEK 9

Day	Workout	Conditions	Comments
1	6 miles		
2	8 miles		
3	10 miles*		
4	6 miles		
5	4 miles		
6	8 miles (race of 5–6-mile distance)		
7			

Daily avg.:

Mileage for week:

_____

_____

_____

*See Notes, p. 172.

If you must run on busy roads, face traffic; run on the left-hand side of the road. Run close to the curb, and if possible, run on the sidewalk. Runners prefer asphalt to all other surfaces or at least find it more convenient. One reason may be that asphalt is more shock absorbent and easier on the feet than the concrete of which most sidewalks are made.

PROGRAM PROCEDURES: TEN-KILOMETER RACE

STAGE 3R: WEEK 10

Day	Workout	Conditions	Comments
1	8 miles		
2	6 miles		
3	10 miles**		
4	8 miles		
5	8 miles		
6	10 miles*		
7			

Daily avg.:

Mileage for week:

*See Notes, p. 172.
**See Notes, p. 172.

The outer layer of clothes is your wind protection and should consist of a light windbreaker jacket in a fabric that "breathes," such as nylon. This outer layer controls heat loss by convection. To regulate heat, you can unzip it or easily remove it and either pocket it or tie it around your waist.

PROGRAM PROCEDURES: TEN-KILOMETER RACE

STAGE 3R: WEEK 11

Day	Workout	Conditions	Comments
1	8 miles		
2	6 miles		
3	10 miles*		
4	8 miles		
5	8 miles		
6	10 miles**		
7			

Daily avg.:

Mileage for week:

*See Notes, p. 172.
**See Notes, p. 172.

In hot weather, wear white. Cotton and mesh shirts are superior to nylon in hot weather. In cold weather, wear a light turtleneck shirt. In very cold weather, add loose-fitting long johns and a light pair of mittens or socks.

PROGRAM PROCEDURES: TEN-KILOMETER RACE

STAGE 3R: WEEK 12

Day	Workout	Conditions	Comments
1	8 miles		
2	10 miles		
3	10 miles*		
4	6 miles		
5	4 miles		
6	8 miles (race of 5–6-mile distance)		
7			

Daily avg.:

Mileage for week:

*See Notes, p. 172.

As the days grow shorter, many of us must train either before or after daylight. Safety can thus be an important factor. Use reflective tape (available at hardware stores) on shoes, jacket, etc.

PROGRAM PROCEDURES: TEN-KILOMETER RACE

STAGE 3R: PEAKING WEEK 1

Day	Workout	Conditions	Comments
1	8 miles		
2	6 miles*		
3	10 miles		
4	8 miles		
5	8 miles*		
6	10 miles**		
7			

Daily avg.:

Mileage for week:

Note: The Peaking Week schedules are *not* part of your normal training. You will want to run these programs *only* 2 weeks before a BIG race. It is especially imperative that you concentrate on the quality of your workouts during the peaking stages. Your form should be as close to perfect as possible, and all runs should be performed without stopping to walk. If you can't satisfy those two criteria, you're not ready to try to peak.

*See Notes, p. 172.
**See Notes, p. 172.

Beware of brushing your stopwatch up against another competitor during a race (easy to do in a crowded start). You may accidentally shut off the watch and lose your split times!

PROGRAM PROCEDURES: TEN-KILOMETER RACE

STAGE 3R: PEAKING WEEK 2

Day	Workout	Conditions	Comments
1	8 miles		
2	10 miles		
3	10 miles*		
4	6 miles		
5	4 miles		
6	8 miles (race of 5–6-mile distance)		
7			

Daily avg.:

Mileage for week:

*See Notes, p. 172.

16
STAGE 3F: RUNNING FOR ADVANCED FITNESS (8-week program)

This program is for the fitness runner who wants to move on to a level higher than is attainable by adhering to the schedules in Chapter 13. It requires you to commit 5 days a week to running.

You will have to take better care of—and pay more attention to—yourself as an athlete when you move up to training by this program. Studies find that the incidence of athletic injuries increases noticeably when an athlete starts running more than 30 miles a week. This program takes you over that mark right from Week 1. It also offers fewer days off from running, giving you less time to recover from the accumulating stress.

We're not trying to scare you. Fear creates unconscious physical tension that predisposes you to injury! We're simply apprising you of a fact of athletic life so you may make an informed decision about your training. Running more often, and at higher weekly mileage, means devoting not only more time to the actual running, but also to stretching, sleep, eating, and all other athletic behaviors. An arithmetic increase in the amount of time devoted to exercise results in a geometric increase in the stress on the systems exercised. In plain English, running 10 miles once is a heck of a lot tougher than running 5 miles twice with full recovery between each run. If you want the added fitness, we're all in favor of your going for it—but only if you take proper care of yourself.

PROGRAM PROCEDURES: ADVANCED FITNESS

STAGE 3F: WEEK 1

Day	Workout	Conditions	Comments
1	6 miles		
2	5 miles		
3	8 miles		
4	5 miles		
5	10 miles		
6			
7			

Daily avg.:

Mileage for week:

PROGRAM PROCEDURES: ADVANCED FITNESS

STAGE 3F: WEEK 2

Day	Workout	Conditions	Comments
1	6 miles		
2	5 miles		
3	8 miles		
4	6 miles		
5	10 miles		
6			
7			

Daily avg.:

Mileage for week:

PROGRAM PROCEDURES: ADVANCED FITNESS

STAGE 3F: WEEK 3

Day	Workout	Conditions	Comments
1	6 miles		
2	6 miles		
3	9 miles		
4	6 miles		
6	11 miles		
6			
7			

Daily avg.:

Mileage for week:

PROGRAM PROCEDURES: ADVANCED FITNESS

STAGE 3F: WEEK 4

Day	Workout	Conditions	Comments
1	7 miles		
2	6 miles		
3	9 miles		
4	6 miles		
5	11 miles		
6			
7			

Daily avg.:

Mileage for week:

PROGRAM PROCEDURES: ADVANCED FITNESS

STAGE 3F: WEEK 5

Day	Workout	Conditions	Comments
1	7 miles		
2	6 miles		
3	10 miles		
4	6 miles		
5	12 miles		
6			
7			

Daily avg.:

Mileage for week:

PROGRAM PROCEDURES: ADVANCED FITNESS

STAGE 3F: WEEK 6

Day	Workout	Conditions	Comments
1	6 miles		
2	6 miles		
3	10 miles		
4	6 miles		
5	12 miles		
6			
7			

Daily avg.:

Mileage for week:

PROGRAM PROCEDURES: ADVANCED FITNESS

STAGE 3F: WEEK 7

Day	Workout	Conditions	Comments
1	7 miles		
2	6 miles		
3	10 miles		
4	6 miles		
5	13 miles		
6			
7			

Daily avg.:

Mileage for week:

PROGRAM PROCEDURES: ADVANCED FITNESS

STAGE 3F: WEEK 8

Day	Workout	Conditions	Comments
1	7 miles		
2	6 miles		
3	10 miles		
4	7 miles		
5	13 miles		
6			
7			

Daily avg.:

Mileage for week:

17

STAGE 4R:
TEN-MILE RACE
(12-week program)

This is the first program in which you begin to train as a serious racer. You received a taste of racing in Chapters 14 and 15, which took you through a fun run and a 10-kilometer race. The main goal in a fun run is to go the distance and have a good time doing it. That's still your goal as a more serious racer, but the definition of "fun" becomes more specific: You find it fun to explore your limits of speed and/or endurance. With this training schedule, the long runs get longer and the hard runs get harder. You start putting yourself under considerable athletic stress. This schedule is your first step onto the path of being a racer. Good luck to you!

TRAINING TECHNIQUES

Before you get into any more running activity, there are some terms you should know.

The following are training techniques, not training systems. These techniques can be applied within the systems that have been described, according to the athlete's needs.

Repetition of sprints: The repetition of short sprints is a means of speed preparation for competition. Sprinting means running at maximum speed. Sprinting as a form of training is meant to improve leg power and racing speed.

Slow interval training: This technique develops aerobic endurance. The speed during each workout is faster than in continuous fast running and so adapts the athlete to running with more intense effort. In this type of formal fast-slow running, the heart beats at the rate of approximately 180 beats per minute during the heavy-work phase.

Fast interval training: This technique develops anaerobic endurance or speed endurance. It increases the ability of the runner to withstand fatigue in the absence of an adequate oxygen supply. This method should be used after a basic amount of aerobic endurance has been developed. The heart should beat in excess of 180 times per minute during the work phase.

Repetition running: This technique differs from interval training in terms of the length of each run and the degree of recovery following each effort. It involves repetitions of comparatively longer distances with relatively complete recovery after each effort, during which time the heart rate reduces to below 120 beats per minute. Repetition running involves distances of half a mile to two miles. Conversely, interval training usually includes repetitions of shorter distances (110 to 660 yards) with less complete recovery after each effort.

Interval sprinting: The athlete sprints about 50 yards, then jogs 20 yards, and repeats the intervals up to three times. After the few sprints, fatigue tends to inhibit the athlete from running at top speed. Similarly, fatigue causes the athlete to reduce recovery jogging to a very slow pace.

Acceleration sprinting: This technique involves acceleration from jogging to striding to sprinting. For example, an athlete may jog 25 yards, stride 50 yards, sprint 50 yards, and then walk 60 yards. The process may be repeated several times. This type of training emphasizes both speed and endurance, provided enough repetitions are performed to cause endurance overload.

Long Sprints: This technique consists of two sprints joined by a recovery jogging. Examples include sprint 50, jog 50, and walk 50 yards for recovery prior to repetition; sprint 110, jog 110, sprint 110, and walk 110 yards before repetition; sprint 220, jog 220, sprint 220, and walk 220 yards before repeating.

What are workouts doing?

1. Sprint workouts and fast interval workouts are for speed.
2. Slow interval workouts and continuous runs increase endurance.
3. Pace interval, repetition runs, and stress workouts improve pace.

ANAEROBIC TRAINING

For distance races, the physiological importance of the aerobic mechanism of the body increases with the distance run. In all races, however, the importance of the anaerobic mechanism of the body should not be overlooked. Whether it is coping with a racing pace that is faster than the athlete's "steady state," or being able to sprint at the finish, it is obvious that the athlete should consider the most efficient method of developing this quality.

Research on anaerobic energy sources indicates that the trained person is generally able to withstand a higher lactic acid concentration than the untrained one. Whether this difference is due to physiological changes or merely a greater ability of the athlete to withstand the associated pain as a result of training is open to conjecture. In any case, it does seem to argue against the case of drawing an arbitrary line in training between the development of the two types of endurance (aerobic and anaerobic).

There are a number of types of training available for enhancing the anaerobic capability of the distance runner. One of the more effective methods to increase the ability to withstand lactic acid build-up is as follows: the athlete runs at maximal effort and then repeats the procedure three or four times. This type of training causes glycogen to break down into lactic acid, and at the end of such a training session the athlete should approach maximal or near-maximal levels of lactic acid concentration in the blood. The highest

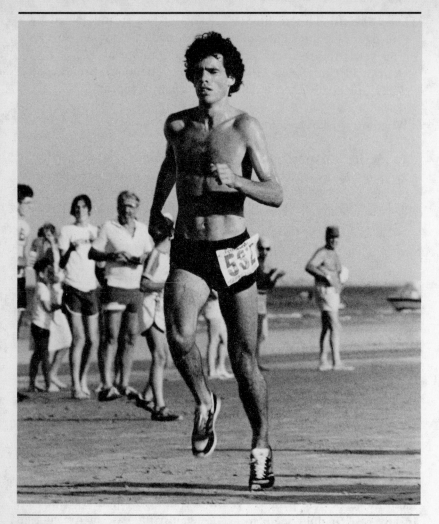

Midway through a summer race, Vin Flemming demonstrates proper arm carriage and knee lift to maintain a sustained, but not sprinting, pace. (Photograph by Bill Boyle)

recorded values for blood lactate concentration have come from athletes who have completed a long-distance run occasionally of over 880 yards.

It should be stressed that even almost pure aerobic training has a beneficial training effort on the anaerobic functioning of the body; however, the greater the intensity of the running, the greater the anaerobic training. In addition, for anaerobic training to be as effective as possible, it should be directed to those muscle groups that will actually be used for fast running. More will be said of this factor later.

INTERVAL TRAINING

A scientific breakthrough by Woldemar Gerschler, famous coach from Freiberg University, and Dr. Reindell, a cardiologist, was the discovery that the heart is the key to endurance performance and, therefore, is virtually the only organ worth worrying about. Briefly, they found that raising the heart to approximately its maximum number of beats per minute (about 180) by running a set distance and then having a recovery period (not to exceed 90 seconds) in order to bring the pulse rate back to 120 beats per minute caused the heart to enlarge during the *recovery phase,* when the pulse rate dropped from 180 to 120 beats per minute. This being the case, they reasoned that the more times this happened, the greater the training effect. Thus, running repeat distances of 100, 220, 330 yards are used.

While an athlete's maximal oxygen uptake is a significant measurement for the distance runner, also of great importance is the amount of time he can maintain his oxygen uptake at a maximal level. Training enables the runner to perform at maximal oxygen uptake level for a longer time than would otherwise be possible. Other factors to consider here are motivation, the resistance of the athlete to pain, the employment of long runs in a "steady state" (in which oxygen uptake balances the oxygen requirement for continuation of effort). The general trend since the 1970s seems to favor this method over pure interval training as a means of attaining and preserving maximal oxygen uptake. Long, slow distance is effective via continuous runs with a pulse rate of about 130 beats per minute at a slow enough pace to avoid lactic acid build-up. This form of training will enable the athlete to improve maximal aerobic power while performing at a fraction of that level for a considerable time. The alternative is to train at a level closer to the maximal, but for a necessarily shorter time.

To train at maximal levels of oxygen uptake, athletes have a number of options open to them. They may carry out a number of runs separated by short rest periods. An example would be a series of 440-yard runs at a good steady speed, say, a two-mile pace, with short rest periods between runs. Training of this type requires the body to work at virtually its maximal aerobic power, but with a corresponding increase in lactic acid formation. The same 440-yard runs alternated with longer rest periods will cause the athlete to work below maximal oxygen level, but with a decreased lactic acid build-up.

It is reasonable to assume that since the shorter rest method more nearly approaches the conditions experienced in a race, it may prove more beneficial. After all, you should be training to work as hard as possible for a given time (the time taken for the race) rather than to recover as quickly as possible from a given number of short efforts.

A method involving longer work periods at submaximal effort is a more efficient method of improving maximal oxygen uptake. This method involves runs separated by rests or easy jogging for a similar length of time and is based on the premise that it is not necessary to delve into anaerobic sources of energy supply for attaining maximal oxygen uptake. To explain this concept further, let us take the case of an athlete running 880 yards. Should he run this course to exhaustion, his maximal oxygen uptake will be unable to supply his full oxygen requirement. He will have to fall back on his anaerobic reserves. However, by running at a slower pace, the athlete can still exercise his maximal oxygen uptake to the full while not accumulating very high oxygen debt. It is suggested, then, that training for maximal oxygen uptake perhaps might take the form of running medium-paced efforts separated by one-half distance jobs. A speed that is 80 percent of maximum has been suggested. The speed should be set according to the experience of the athlete. A sufficient guideline is to run at a speed that does not cause acute ventilation problems.

TIPS ON WEATHER: ADVICE FOR THE RUNNER

1. If wind speed is 15 mph and temperature 30°F, the effective temperature is 10°F. At this temperature there is increasing danger of frostbite, and protective measures should be taken.
2. To date, the best and cheapest remedy for a cold seems to be moderate amounts of aspirin, liquids, and plenty of rest.

3. If your feet are cold, put on a hat. The head radiates more heat than any other part of the body. At 40°F (without a hat), you can lose up to one-half of the body's total heat production. At 5°F, you lose three-quarters of body heat. It is not your clothes that keep you warm, it's the air in your clothes. Air forms an insulating layer that keeps the body heat inside.

4. In cold weather dress properly. Wear thermal underwear, heavy sweaters, hood and face mask, mittens, and something around the neck. Wearing these clothes, running during the warmer part of the day (between 1 P.M. and 4 P.M.), and running where the environment breaks the wind make cold-weather running a lot easier.

5. Make sure your clothing is wind-proof and inner clothing is loose. Tight-fitting clothing cuts off the circulation and increases the danger of freezing.

6. All the experts agree that frostbite victims should not use ice or hot water on the affected area. Gradually rewarm the area with water that is nearly body temperature and seek medical help immediately.

7. In hot weather, run in light clothing, and wear a brimmed hat that gives shade to your face in the sun. In addition, run at the cooler times of the day: early morning or evening. Beat the heat, not yourself. The guidelines are simple:
   a. Take an hour a day of increasing activity for two weeks to acclimate to heat.
   b. Take fluid often and early, every twenty minutes.
   c. Take fluids with adequate electrolytes, such as ERG.
   d. Increasing fluids combined with decreasing activity is the best protection. Acknowledge danger signals and cancel practice or competition, if necessary.

PROGRAM PROCEDURES: TEN-MILE RACE

STAGE 4R: WEEK 1

Day	Workout	Conditions	Comments
1	8 miles		
2	10 miles		
3	8 miles		
4	10 miles*		
5	8 miles		
6	12 miles		
7			

Daily avg.:

Mileage for week:

*See Notes, p. 172.

Try to find some enjoyable running companions for long runs. Many times company and comradeship get you through workouts that otherwise you might have missed.

PROGRAM PROCEDURES: TEN-MILE RACE

STAGE 4R: WEEK 2

Day	Workout	Conditions	Comments
1	8 miles		
2	10 miles**		
3	8 miles		
4	10 miles		
5	8 miles		
6	12 miles		
7			

Daily avg.:

Mileage for week:

** See Notes, p. 172.

Flexibility Test 1

Try to follow tests. If you fail them, you're tight:
    With knees unbent, touch your palms to the floor.
    Stand with heels together and see if knees bend backward twenty degrees or more.
    Keep stretching.

PROGRAM PROCEDURES: TEN-MILE RACE

STAGE 4R: WEEK 3

Day	Workout	Conditions	Comments
1	8 miles		
2	10 miles		
3	10 miles*		
4	8 miles		
5	4 miles		
6	12 miles (race 10–12-mile distance)		
7			

Daily avg.:

Mileage for week:

_____

_____

_____

_____

*See Notes, p. 172.

You don't have time not to warm up and down properly. The price of success is the proper work for you and your body.

PROGRAM PROCEDURES: TEN-MILE RACE

STAGE 4R: WEEK 4

Day	Workout	Conditions	Comments
1	8 miles		
2	10 miles*		
3	8 miles		
4	10 miles		
5	8 miles*		
6	12 miles		
7			

Daily avg.:

Mileage for week:

*See Notes, p. 172.
On the long run, time the first half of the run and retrace the distance at slightly faster tempo. Do not try to race distance or push yourself too hard.

Flexibility Test 2

Hold arms out straight with palms up so that the little fingers are higher than the thumbs.
   Sit or lie down comfortably in the lotus position.
   Turn feet out 90°.
Keep stretching.

PROGRAM PROCEDURES: TEN-MILE RACE

STAGE 4R: WEEK 5

Day	Workout	Conditions	Comments
1	8 miles		
2	10 miles		
3	8 miles**		
4	12 miles		
5	10 miles		
6	12 miles		
7			

Daily avg.:

Mileage for week:

**See Notes, p. 172.

A money-saving tip for preserving the heels of track shoes is to place two strips of athletic tape across the heel. This timely trick adds several miles of wear. Many tendon strains are caused by worn heels.

PROGRAM PROCEDURES: TEN-MILE RACE

STAGE 4R: WEEK 6

Day	Workout	Conditions	Comments
1	8 miles		
2	10 miles*		
3	8 miles		
4	12 miles		
5	10 miles**		
6	12 miles		
7			

Daily avg.:

Mileage for week:

*See Notes, p. 172.
**See Notes, p. 172.

Plan three running courses to relieve boredom, for variety is the spice of life.

PROGRAM PROCEDURES: TEN-MILE RACE

STAGE 4R: WEEK 7

Day	Workout	Conditions	Comments
1	8 miles		
2	10 miles*		
3	12 miles		
4	8 miles		
5	6 miles*		
6	12 miles		
7			

Daily avg.:

Mileage for week:

_____

_____

_____

_____

*See Notes, p. 172.

At finish, all distance runners become sprinters. Each week incorporate sprint pick-ups in the training program on the run.

PROGRAM PROCEDURES: TEN-MILE RACE

STAGE 4R: WEEK 8

Day	Workout	Conditions	Comments
1	8 miles		
2	10 miles*		
3	8 miles		
4	12 miles		
5	10 miles**		
6	12 miles		
7			

Daily avg.:

Mileage for week:

*See Notes, p. 172.
**See Notes, p. 172.

Wear training shoes that are not drastically different from your racing shoes. This rule is quite important because of the amount of heel raise. If you train in a high heel wedge and race in a flat shoe, considerable fatigue is sure to develop.

PROGRAM PROCEDURES: TEN-MILE RACE

STAGE 4R: WEEK 9

Day	Workout	Conditions	Comments
1	10 miles		
2	10 miles*		
3	8 miles		
4	12 miles		
5	8 miles**		
6	14 miles		
7			

Daily avg.:

Mileage for week:

*See Notes, p. 172.
**See Notes, p. 172.

The value of hill running is that it builds speed, strength, knee lift, leg strength, and leg stride. Find a gradual hill with a 440-to-600-yard length so that you may run down safely and your body will adapt to strain.

PROGRAM PROCEDURES: TEN-MILE RACE

STAGE 4R: WEEK 10

Day	Workout	Conditions	Comments
1	10 miles		
2	10 miles*		
3	8 miles		
4	12 miles		
5	8 miles**		
6	14 miles		
7			

Daily avg.:

Mileage for week:

*See Notes, p. 172.
**See Notes, p. 172.

When running uphill, lean slightly forward, drop your hands a little, pump them harder, and concentrate on lifting your knees.

When running downhill, hold your hands higher and relax. Let gravity pull you downhill and feel relaxed.

PROGRAM PROCEDURES: TEN-MILE RACE

STAGE 4R: WEEK 11

Day	Workout	Conditions	Comments
1	10 miles		
2	8 miles		
3	14 miles*		
4	10 miles		
5	6 miles		
6	12 miles (race of 10–12 miles)		
7			

Daily avg.:

Mileage for week:

*See Notes, p. 172.

Watch your form for excessive up and down motion and twisting action. You need to think a lot about style as fatigue mounts. Have a friend take your picture on the run and note your flaws.

PROGRAM PROCEDURES: TEN-MILE RACE

STAGE 4R: WEEK 12

Day	Workout	Conditions	Comments
1	10 miles		
2	10 miles		
3	8 miles**		
4	12 miles		
5	8 miles		
6	14 miles		
7			

Daily avg.:

Mileage for week:

**See Notes, p. 172.

It is necessary to reiterate the description of the overuse syndrome and to stress the importance of keeping the bodily systems in balance. Overextension will result in physical injury, so runners must learn their bodily limitations.

PROGRAM PROCEDURES: TEN-MILE RACE

STAGE 4R: PEAKING WEEK 1

Day	Workout	Conditions	Comments
1	10 miles		
2	8 miles		
3	14 miles*		
4	10 miles		
5	6 miles		
6	12 miles**		
7			

Daily avg.:

Mileage for week:

*See Notes, p. 172.
**See Notes, p. 172.

Note: The Peaking Week schedules are *not* part of your normal training. You will want to run these programs *only* 2 weeks before a BIG race. It is especially imperative that you concentrate on the quality of your workouts during the peaking stages. Your form should be as close to perfect as possible, and all runs should be performed without stopping to walk. If you can't satisfy those two criteria, you're not ready to try to peak.

Should I Run Double Workouts?

No, not until you're running more mileage than recommended by any training program in this book. Exercise physiologists have found that a two-hour run gives 120 percent of the training benefits of two one-hour runs.

PROGRAM PROCEDURES: TEN-MILE RACE

STAGE 4R: PEAKING WEEK 2

Day	Workout	Conditions	Comments
1	8 miles		
2	10 miles*		
3	8 miles		
4	6 miles		
5	4 miles		
6	Race		
7			

Daily avg.:

Mileage for week:

*See Notes, p. 172.

18

STAGE 5: EMERGENCY MAINTENANCE PROGRAM

It sometimes happens that you are unable to run your normal training schedule. Most runners worry about losing their fitness at such times. This training program will help you lose as little aerobic fitness as possible while also allowing you the time to tend to the more mundane demands of your life.

We must, however, stress that this is an emergency program. It is not a program by which you can train week after week. It will help you lose as little fitness as possible, but you *will* decline the more you stay on the program. That is why the program lasts only 4 weeks. After that, you must accept a lower level of fitness, and when you go back to your normal training, resume it at a more elementary pace than where you left it. No one enjoys it when circumstances force a fitness decline, but remember that running is your hobby, not your life. You'll regain your lost fitness. We all do.

You'll notice that the program provides no specific mileage or other instructions. You'll have to figure that out for yourself. The program instructions are simple. A mileage instruction such as "average daily distance" means that, for that day, you run the number of miles you've been averaging per day on your normal training program. For example, if you've been sticking with Week 12 of the Basic Fitness Program, you've been running 25 miles a week on a 4-day schedule, resulting in a daily average mileage of 6.25.

Begin the program with either Week 1 or Week 2. If you've been running 5 or more days a week and have the time, start with Week 1. If you've been running 4 days a week, and/or are really pressed for running time, start with Week 2. Stay on the program as short a time as possible to avoid fitness decline.

Runners following the racing programs will notice there are no hill sessions or speed pick-up runs indicated in this schedule. Do such runs as you see fit. If you feel up to hill repeats, do them. The same with pick-ups. Don't *force* yourself to do either of these anaerobic sessions. In this kind of emergency maintenance program, your mileage is much more important. It's the base on which your anaerobic workouts depend.

You need not run these workouts one day after the other. You should follow the daily instructions in the order given, but you may miss days in between workouts. Just get in the outlined workouts every week.

A special note on Week 3, Day 3: Here you add 1 to 2 miles to the longest distance you run when following your normal program. If your weekly long run is 8 miles, you would run 9 or 10 miles on this day. In general, fitness runners will want to add 1 mile, and racers will add 2 miles. But the bottom line here is to run what feels good. If your body tells you that an extra mile is plenty, listen to it.

PROGRAM PROCEDURES: EMERGENCY MAINTENANCE

STAGE 5: WEEK 1

Day	Workout	Conditions	Comments
1	average daily distance		
2	second-longest normal weekly run		
3	average daily distance		
4	longest normal weekly run		
5			
6			
7			

Daily avg.:

Mileage for week:

PROGRAM PROCEDURES: EMERGENCY MAINTENANCE

STAGE 5: WEEK 2

Day	Workout	Conditions	Comments
1	average daily distance		
2	second-longest normal weekly run		
3	longest normal weekly run		
4			
5			
6			
7			

Daily avg.:

Mileage for week:

PROGRAM PROCEDURES: EMERGENCY MAINTENANCE

STAGE 5: WEEK 3

Day	Workout	Conditions	Comments
1	second-longest normal weekly run		
2	average daily distance		
3	longest normal weekly run plus 1 to 2 miles		
4			
5			
6			
7			

Daily avg.: _____

Mileage for week: _____

_____

_____

_____

_____

PROGRAM PROCEDURES: EMERGENCY MAINTENANCE

STAGE 5: WEEK 4

Day	Workout	Conditions	Comments
1	longest normal weekly run		
2	jog 20 minutes		
3	jog 20 minutes		
4	longest normal weekly run		
5			
6			
7			

Daily avg.: _____

Mileage for week: _____

_____

_____

_____

_____

19

STAGE 6R:
MARATHON BASE
(8-week program)

This is a competition training program that helps you build enough strength to begin training to race a marathon. (The marathon race training schedule itself is in the following chapter.) You'll notice that this program requires you to run nearly every day. Some of the running days are optional, as noted in the schedule charts. If you feel you need the rest, then take that optional day off. You will nonetheless be making a serious time commitment if you enter this program and the one in Chapter 20.

Training to race a marathon requires a serious commitment because racing a marathon is a serious matter. The marathon base and race programs will help you realize your fullest potential in competing in a marathon. If you haven't the time or motivation to follow these programs, that does not reflect badly on you as an athlete. It only means that you should not race a marathon. Nowhere is it written that a person is not a runner until he or she has raced a marathon. Even if you've the time and motivation, you may find your body complains at the high mileage. If so, listen to it. Train at shorter distances and be healthy and happy.

If you don't have the time or talent to follow these programs but still want to run (instead of race) a marathon, you'll find the program you want in our book *Improving Women's Running*. In fact, many athletes of both sexes have used the Marathon Run Program

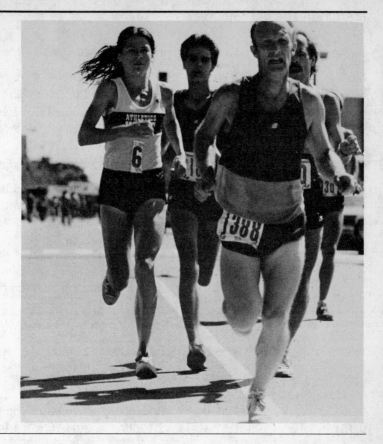

Most marathoners, as well as short-distance runners, run in packs during a race for mutual support; it is, therefore, important for runners in training to run with others. (Photograph by Bill Boyle)

in that book to help them prepare for the marathon racing programs in this one.

CARDIAC CONCERNS: MAXIMUM HEART RATE

Maximum heart rate is a function of age. It has nothing to do with fitness. A rule of thumb, which is subject to great variation, is that the figure 220 minus your age gives you your maximum heart rate. No matter how hard you exercise, your heart can beat no faster. It is intrinsic within the heart's ability to beat and has nothing to do with

Marathon Pacing Guide

1 Mile	5 Miles	10 Miles	15 Miles	20 Miles	Marathon
6:00	30:00	1:00:00	1:30:00	2:00:00	2:37:10
6:10	30:50	1:01:40	1:32:30	2:03:20	2:41:41
6:20	31:40	1:03:20	1:35:00	2:06:40	2:46:03
6:30	32:30	1:05:00	1:37:30	2:10:00	2:50:25
6:40	33:20	1:06:40	1:40:00	2:13:20	2:54:47
6:50	34:10	1:08:20	1:42:30	2:16:40	2:59:09
7:00	35:00	1:10:00	1:45:00	2:20:00	3:03:33
7:10	35:00	1:11:40	1:18:20	2:23:20	3:07:55
7:20	36:40	1:13:20	1:50:00	2:26:40	3:12:17
7:30	37:30	1:15:00	1:52:30	2:30:00	3:16:39
7:40	38:20	1:16:40	1:55:00	2:33:20	3:21:01
7:50	39:10	1:18:20	1:57:30	2:36:40	3:25:23
8:00	40:00	1:20:00	2:00:00	2:40:00	3:29:46
8:10	40:30	1:21:40	2:02:30	2:43:20	3:34:08
8:20	41:40	1:23:20	2:05:00	2:46:40	3:38:30
8:30	42:30	1:25:00	2:07:30	2:50:00	3:42:52
8:40	43:20	1:26:40	2:10:00	2:53:20	3:47:14
8:50	44:10	1:28:20	2:12:30	2:56:40	3:51:36
9:00	45:00	1:30:00	2:15:00	3:00:00	3:56:00
9:10	45:50	1:31:40	2:17:30	3:03:20	4:00:22

Marathon Per-Mile Pace

World best:	4:50.5—2:07	6:10—2:41:43	7:40—3:21:01
American best:	4:53—2:08	6:20—2:46:03	7:50—3:25:23
	5:00—2:11:06	6:30—2:50:25	8:00—3:29:46
	5:10—2:15:28	6:40—2:54:47	8:10—3:34:08
	5:20—2:19:50	6:50—2:59:09	8:20—3:38:30
	5:30—2:24:12	7:00—3:03:32	8:30—3:42:52
	5:40—2:28:34	7:10—3:07:54	8:40—3:47:14
	5:50—2:32:56	7:20—3:12:16	8:50—3:51:36
	6:00—2:37:19	7:30—3:16:39	9:00—3:56:00

Distance Race Measurements

3000 meters	=	1 mile, 1521 yds.
5000 meters	=	3 miles, 189 yds.
10,000 meters	=	6 miles, 378 yds.
15 kilometers	=	9 miles, 565 yds.
20 kilometers	=	12 miles, 755 yds.
30 kilometers	=	18 miles, 1130 yds.
Marathon	=	26 miles, 385 yds.
50 kilometers	=	31 miles, 121 yds.

fitness. There is tremendous variation in heart rate. For example, one young adult's maximum heart rate may be generally about 196 beats per minute, but a group of young adults in relatively the same condition can have maximum rates between 170 and 215 beats per minute.

The goal eventually is to exercise strenuously enough to achieve 70 percent of the maximum expected heart rate for twenty to thirty minutes, three or four times per week. (This percentage of the maximum expected heart rate can vary as much as ±20, depending on the condition of the individual.)

Another popular indicator of a person's level of fitness is the heart rate at rest, measured in terms of beats per minute. The more fit an individual is, the fewer times the heart beats per minute at rest. This phenomenon is due to the fact that the heart, like any other muscle, becomes stronger and more efficient with continued exercise. Thus, it can pump a greater volume of blood with each beat. The lower the resting heart rate, the better the level of conditioning.

WHAT WILL YOU HAVE TO DRINK?

If your practice runs are six miles and longer, you might want to try six ounces of grape juice and the same amount of water. Grape juice has a higher natural sugar level and a higher glucose level than other juices and contains a lot of electrolytes (minerals). You need the glucose for energy and the electrolytes to replace what you lose while you sweat.

Liquid nourishment is a must when you're running six miles or more each day. You can dehydrate the kidneys if you don't take in some liquid nourishment—preferably the water and grape-juice mixture—before you run.

Should athletes drink tea or coffee twenty-four hours before a race? Many athletes ordinarily do drink tea and coffee. In the past, tea has been traditionally a part of the precompetition meal. The caffeine in tea induces a period of stimulation of the central nervous system followed by a period of depression. Since the athlete is usually excited and nervous during the period immediately preceding competition, the addition of caffeine to the last meal may not be advisable and may increase nervousness. The same caution applies to coffee. Both tea and coffee are diuretics; that is, they stimulate the flow of urine. Thus, they may cause additional discomfort during the competitive period.

Coffee and tea both contain about 1–5 grains of caffeine per cup, and they stimulate the heart, nerves, and kidneys. The choice to drink or not to drink is yours.

Facts you should know about caffeine. The bottom line is that caffeine is a drug. Caffeine is an alkaline substance. Caffeine drinks are used for their stimulant effect as well as for their flavor. They cause the heart and lungs to work at an abnormally fast rate.

Under the influence of caffeine, the kidneys excrete more fluid than normal and the stomach secretes more acid. Individuals who consume lots of caffeine urinate more than other people and frequently have heartburn.

Caffeine also stimulates the body to release sugar into the blood stream. Increasing blood sugar depresses the appetite, but the effect is temporary. When the concentration of blood sugar falls, hunger returns. Taking more caffeine (in coffee, for example) increases blood sugar again, and so on. Some diets prohibit caffeine drinks to prevent the roller-coaster effects of high-low-high blood sugar.

Amounts of caffeine in beverages are not consistent. Some coffees and teas are higher in caffeine than others. The method by which the beverage is prepared is a factor relating to caffeine content. A premedical student at Columbia University measured the amounts

Caffeine Contents of Popular Beverages

	Caffeine Content
Tea—bag	46 mg
Coffee—ground	85 mg
Coca-Cola (can or bottle)	24 mg
Pepsi-Cola (can or bottle)	18 mg
Cocoa (can or jar)	50 mg
Sanka (can or jar)	3.3 mg
Nestlé Decaf (can or jar)	0.18 mg

Note: "Stay-awake" pills contain 100 milligrams of caffeine. Headache and cold preparations contain about 30 milligrams.

of caffeine in teas brewed different ways. The report of the study said that tea made with loose leaves yields more caffeine than tea made in bags. Iced tea has more caffeine than hot tea. The accompanying chart shows some of the test results for tea and other beverages. All teas were made by steeping the leaves in hot water for four minutes in a six-ounce cup.

If caffeine is a problem for you, taper off slowly. Switch from a high-caffeine beverage to one that contains less caffeine, and cut down on the number of cups of it per day.

Alcohol

The use of alcohol cannot be justified or recommended. In small quantities (such as found in beer), alcohol affects the finer neuromuscular coordinations. In large quantities, it affects gross coordination to a considerable degree. Tolerance of alcohol by the human machine requires energy that cannot be divided between muscular effort and the oxidation of alcohol. The liver plays an important role in athletics with regard to the conversion of protein into carbohydrates in the process of gluconeogenesis. Thus liver damage resulting from alcohol consumption is an important issue in athletic performance. During exercise, the liver must convert lactic acid back into liver glycogen, in a circuit known as the *Corci cycle*. Liver tissue forms glycogen from simple sugar, and the liver serves as the storehouse for glycogen. The brain and heart are the chief users of glycogen. Obviously, well-trained athletes can perform at highest efficiency only if their reserves of sugar are not molested by such irritations as the oxidation of alcohol, which robs the liver of its elasticity and tone. Over a long period of athletic stress the liver cannot be expected to render efficient service to both the muscles and alcohol oxidation. Mixing alcohol and athletics is comparable to burning the candle at both ends. It is now known that even small amounts of beer adversely affect the body's heat regulatory mechanism for twenty-four to twenty-eight hours.

Water

The best thing you can drink is water. The body absorbs water more quickly than it absorbs any other thirst-quenching fluid, and (if the water is room temperature) with no possible negative side-effects. There is no other drink about which that statement can be made, according to David Costill of the Ball State University human performance laboratory.

The best thing for the athlete to drink *before, during, and after* exercise (especially competition) is water. Forget the so-called fluid replacement drinks. If you're eating a balanced diet, you are getting all the electrolyte and mineral replacement you need.

Some drinks are positively harmful to the dehydrated athlete. These are drinks that have a diuretic effect (drinks that contain alcohol or caffeine—something like Irish coffee would be the worst possible drink you could take after a workout!).

Extremely dry air is another problem for the dehydration-fighter. The traveling athlete should note, then, that the air in a commercial airliner's passenger cabin is exceptionally dry and circulates rapidly, sucking away your precious sweat. If you've just flown in for a race—never a smart idea, but sometimes unavoidable—drink even more water than you normally would before the gun sounds.

You may assume such advice is superfluous. "I'll drink until I'm not thirsty," you're probably thinking. "I'll naturally compensate if I'm flight-parched. My mouth will stay dry until I've reestablished visceral equilibrium." Unfortunately, you very well may not. Your sense of thirst is not an accurate index of your degree of hydration.

Thirst can be "quenched" by ingesting only one-third to one-half the water necessary to restore what has been sweated away. There are three handy indices of the adequacy of your water intake: (1) Your weight: what goes out must go back in; keep drinking until you weigh as much after the run as you did before it. (2) Your urine: if it's extremely dark, it's too concentrated, and you need to drink more water. (Some problems will arise with this index if one is an advanced athlete who puts in a lot of high quality workouts. Dark urine may indicate high levels of lactic acid build-up—perfectly normal when doing quality work—and it may also be attributable to small quantities of blood in the urine—which is also perfectly normal and *no* cause for alarm.) (3) Your strength: you'll know within a few days if you're not drinking enough, because you'll be weak and/or dead. If you find this last index unpleasant, pay close attention to the first and second indices instead.

Start drinking your water two hours before a race. Medical authorities suggest consuming around thirty-eight ounces of water during this period, but you will have to experiment to determine what is best for you personally. You might want to experiment with drinking three eight-ounce glasses within 2 hours before the race. If you weight around 90 pounds, for example, chugging a quart of H_2O before the race will have you swimming across the line, looking for the nearest Porta-John. Perhaps the best rule of thumb is to keep drinking until you're no longer thirsty, then drink some more.

It is vitally important that you drink *during* the race; you should therefore practice taking drinks from tiny, soggy, paper cups during your training runs, so you won't have to slow down or stop during a big race. In racing, it is mandatory to take water early and often. Don't plan on taking one big drink at the halfway mark in any race, even a 10K. It is far more physiologically efficient to take a lot of little drinks than one big one.

Finally, when racing, don't forget that water has a salutory effect on performance when applied externally as well as when drunk. Remember what a little heat-radiator your head is (which is why you keep warm in the winter by wearing a wool cap and little else). Help your head radiate heat by soaking it with water during the race—but beware of getting your feet wet, unless you like running on blisters (which is why it's a good idea to stay away from well-meaning but often "aimless" spectators who offer to douse you with their garden hose).

CARBOHYDRATE LOADING: PROS AND CONS

The concept of carbohydrate loading was developed by a Swedish physiologist. According to the theory, if the glycogen stored in the muscle cells is depleted and then replaced suddenly, the muscles tend to overload so that glycogen stores become significantly greater than at normal resting levels. This increased supply of glycogen should give a runner extra energy and strength for the latter part of a long endurance race such as a marathon.

The carbohydrate-loading technique takes seven days. So, preparing for a Sunday race, you would begin the training program the previous Sunday so that day 7 would fall on Saturday, the day before the race. The procedure is as follows:

Day 1: Take a long run, approximately eighteen to twenty miles, to deplete the glycogen reserves in the muscles.

Days 2, 3, and 4: Train a bit below your normal routine and eat a diet high in protein and very low in carbohydrates. The depletion part of the carbohydrate-loading schedule puts a great deal of stress on the body. You may experience moments of fatigue and become very irritable at this time.

Days 5, 6, and 7: Train very lightly and eat a high-carbohydrate diet. It is very tempting to overeat during this part of the schedule. To avoid any weight gain, maintain your normal caloric intake. On the day of the race it is very important to be well rested, so get eight hours of sleep the night before. The additional packing of glycogen at this time is minimal since there is not enough time for these additional carbohydrates to metabolize. Also, any undigested food that may be stored in your stomach at the start of the race could be detrimental to your performance.

It is important to monitor yourself very carefully because there is some danger of hypoglycemia, or low blood sugar, during the training period of the week preceding the competition. Symptoms of hypoglycemia are dizziness and fainting. Extreme weakness usually results during the low-carbohydrate phase, so during this period you ought to limit your training to approximately half, without any long or strenuous runs, to avoid excessive fatigue. During the second phase of the diet, it is important to limit the amount of running you do so that the glycogen, which is building slowly, is not depleted prior to the race.

Performed properly, the carbohydrate-loading "diet" definitely seems beneficial in efforts over twenty miles, but it requires careful monitoring and guarantees no definite results. At the 1976 Olympic trials, only five athletes used loading and those athletes did not qualify for the Olympic squad.

Loading Has Problems

Let's say a race is Sunday. On Monday, Tuesday, and Wednesday a runner eats no carbohydrates. Then on Thursday, Friday, and Saturday, the runner consumes carbohydrates such as breads, potatoes, and pastas. The theory is that depletion, followed by loading, enables the body to pack more carbohydrates than it normally would be able to hold.

The process is tiring for the body. The increase of sugar in the bloodstream triggers a momentary burst of energy, but it is followed by the production of insulin, which lowers the blood sugar and decreases energy.

Besides the high-low cycle, there is a second factor to consider: some say that carbohydrates consumed days before a race won't be available to the body when they are needed. They will have turned to fat, which will be of little use in the race. So add a few extra carbohydrates the day before the race for usable fuel.

PROGRAM PROCEDURES: MARATHON BASE

STAGE 6R: WEEK 1

Day	Workout	Conditions	Comments
1	8 miles		
2	12 miles		
3	6 miles		
4	10 miles**		
5	8 miles		
6	16 miles		
7			

Daily avg.:

Mileage for week:

**See Notes, p. 172.

During a race, ice cubes are a very good addition to a water station. They can be rubbed on the back of the neck, the underside of your wrists, and on your forehead to lower body temperature, and they provide an additional source of water. Likewise, getting dowsed with a hose not only feels good, it can safeguard your health, but do not allow wetting the chest area.

PROGRAM PROCEDURES: MARATHON BASE

STAGE 6R: WEEK 2

Day	Workout	Conditions	Comments
1	8 miles		
2	12 miles		
3	6 miles or day off		
4	8 miles		
5	10 miles**		
6	8 miles		
7	16 miles		

Daily avg.:

Mileage for week:

**See Notes, p. 172.

Warm down after vigorous activity to allow the muscles to dissipate the waste products (lactic acid). Get legs up!

PROGRAM PROCEDURES: MARATHON BASE

STAGE 6R: WEEK 3

Day	Workout	Conditions	Comments
1	8 miles		
2	12 miles		
3	6 miles		
4	10 miles*		
5	8 miles		
6	8 miles		
7	16 miles (race 10–18-mile distance)		

Daily avg.:

Mileage for week:

*See Notes, p. 172.

Review results of race tactics, analyze your strengths and weaknesses. Work on improving both.

  There should be no weak links in your physical chain.

PROGRAM PROCEDURES: MARATHON BASE

STAGE 6R: WEEK 4

Day	Workout	Conditions	Comments
1	8 miles		
2	12 miles**		
3	6 miles or day off		
4	8 miles		
5	10 miles*		
6	8 miles		
7	16 miles		

Daily avg.:

Mileage for week:

*See Notes, p. 172.
**See Notes, p. 172.

During a race, if you feel winded or light-headed, rest until you're in control again. If you get a stitch in your side, slow down, take deep breaths, dangle your arms at your sides, and concentrate on keeping the upper portion of your body relaxed. Drink a small amount of fluid at each aid station.

PROGRAM PROCEDURES: MARATHON BASE

STAGE 6R: WEEK 5

Day	Workout	Conditions	Comments
1	8 miles		
2	10 miles**		
3	12 miles		
4	8 miles or day off		
5	10 miles*		
6	8 miles		
7	16 miles		

Daily avg.:

Mileage for week:

*See Notes, p. 172.
**See Notes, p. 172.

Foot strain usually results when a runner tries to do too much fast running all at once. This injury, like practically all injuries, can be avoided by gradually changing training practices. Allow your body time to adapt to new stresses.

PROGRAM PROCEDURES: MARATHON BASE

STAGE 6R: WEEK 6

Day	Workout	Conditions	Comments
1	8 miles		
2	10 miles*		
3	12 miles		
4	8 miles		
5	8 miles		
6	8 miles		
7	16 miles (race 10–18-mile distance)		

Daily avg.:

Mileage for week:

*See Notes, p. 172.

The two main sources of energy are slow-burning fat stored in muscles (as opposed to excessive fatty tissue common among many Americans) and carbohydrates stored in the muscles and the liver as glycogen. High-carbohydrate diets require 10 percent less oxygen for conversion to energy than protein. Therefore, oxygen is being used more efficiently.

PROGRAM PROCEDURES: MARATHON BASE

STAGE 6R: WEEK 7

Day	Workout	Conditions	Comments
1	8 miles or day off		
2	10 miles**		
3	12 miles		
4	8 miles		
5	10 miles*		
6	8 miles		
7	16 miles		

Daily avg.:

Mileage for week:

*See Notes, p. 172.
**See Notes, p. 172.

The Need for Flex and Weight Work

Training overdevelops the prime movers; it causes the muscles along the back of the leg and thigh and lower back to become short and inflexible. The antagonists, the muscles on the front of the leg and thigh and abdomen, become relatively weak.

PROGRAM PROCEDURES: MARATHON BASE

STAGE 6R: WEEK 8

Day	Workout	Conditions	Comments
1	8 miles		
2	10 miles**		
3	12 miles		
4	8 miles or day off		
5	10 miles		
6	8 miles		
7	16 miles		

Daily avg.:

Mileage for week:

_____

_____

_____

_____

**See Notes, p. 172.

Exercise can help us calm down by normalizing body chemistry. Stress increases the flow of adrenalin, which, if it isn't dissipated by activity, can result in more stress. It may be especially helpful to people prone to depression because "exercise will counter underlying depression if you do it consistently."

20

STAGE 7R:
MARATHON RACE
(18-week program)

The 18 weeks of this training schedule actually constitute an endless loop of a program. Once you have reached this level of fitness, you can continue to run the program over and over, competing in two or three marathons a year. The last 4 weeks of the program help you recover from the marathon. After you've completed the fourth week of the the recovery program (the eighteenth week of the whole schedule), you can turn back to the first week of the program and continue on through the schedule again.

Alternatively, you could cycle back into the last 2 weeks of the Marathon Base Program in the previous chapter. You may well not want to run two or three marathons a year. If that's the case, keep running Weeks 7 and 8 of the Marathon Base Program. That will give you a program allowing you to compete very successfully in all road races shorter than the marathon and will also maintain your fitness to move right back into the Marathon Race Program when and if you want again to prepare for a marathon.

MECHANICS OF FATIGUE

Fatigue has become a socially acceptable excuse for not doing things. It is difficult to measure fatigue or to arrive at its true cause because no two human beings have the same energy resources and because the capacities of individuals vary from day to day. American researchers have spent many years looking for a clue to the mechanics of fatigue. The most intensive studies of fatigue, which were conducted at Harvard University's Fatigue Laboratory, revealed that physical fatigue is caused by a complex chain of chemical reactions. Investigators found that if the human body is to carry a reasonably heavy workload without exhaustion, complete coordination of muscle movements with breathing and circulation is necessary. The muscles rely on glycogen, the energy-producing material for their power to contract; but after prolonged muscular effort, the so-called "fatigue materials"—lactic acid, carbon dioxide, and other by-products—seep into the bloodstream. So acute is the chemical change that injections of blood from a fatigued animal administered to a rested animal will produce fatigue.

Metabolism, regulated by the endocrine glands as their chief function, is the chemical process responsible for the construction of new cells, the destruction of old ones and the rate of release of energy. Of the endocrine glands, the two adrenals, located one over each kidney, are the most reliable aids in rallying the body for the fight against fatigue. The immediate response to heightened emotion—fear, anxiety, and anger—is stepped-up adrenal gland activity. Adrenalin helps the liver to liberate sugar; it also increases the rate and force of the heartbeat and, thereby, the flow of blood into the tired muscles. When spurts of this powerful hormone are released, breathing deepens and the whole body is ready for immediate physical and mental action. In stress studies it was found that the greater the skill, the less the fatigue, and the smaller the runner's increase in adrenal output. The more secure performer calls on his adrenal glands to meet the demands of the situation. This may explain why certain exceptionally gifted people seem tireless.

Endocrine studies also explain the mechanism of the "second wind," that unexpected surge of muscular energy under stress. This increase is caused by the action of the nervous sytem on the adrenal glands. A sudden release of adrenalin into a tired person's blood causes the "second wind" phenomenon.

WHAT TRAINING DOES FOR MUSCLES

The muscles of the lower back and the lower extremities are of prime importance in endurance training. There are three types of

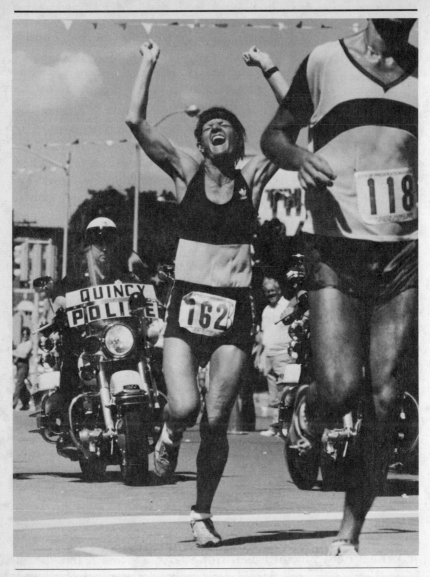

You made it! No matter how many you complete, the marathon finish line is the sweetest sight of all racing, and you deserve to be happy and proud when you cross it. (Photograph by Bill Boyle)

muscles: slow-contracting red-muscle fiber, fast-contracting white fiber, and fast red fiber. For long-distance running, the most important kind is the slow-contracting red-muscle fiber. Generally found deep in the bulk of the muscle, close to the bone, this type has a rich blood supply and is fatigue resistant. These muscles function basically by burning oxygen and what is called *aerobic metabolism*. They are especially important for prolonged effort. Most long-distance runners have a high percentage of these slow aerobic fibers.

The fast-contracting white fiber plays an important role in short, sudden movements; for example, at the start or finish of a race or during hill running. These muscle fibers have a low capacity for oxygen use. Their main energy source is glycogen (carbohydrates). The end-product of their metabolism is lactic acid, so it is these muscle fibers that contribute to lactic acid build-up in muscle fatigue.

The last type of fiber—the fast red fiber—has a good blood supply and is thought to be important for work of relatively high intensity and of some duration. Middle-distance runners have a higher percentage of these particular fibers.

Again, it is important to note that the ultimate energy source necessary for muscle contraction is ATP,* which requires the presence of a certain enzyme within the muscle for its breakdown and use. The fast-contracting fibers, both white and red, contain a high level of these enzymes to break down ATP, whereas the slow red fibers contain lower levels of this particular enzyme. The level of this enzyme in slow red fibers can be markedly increased by endurance training.

Of additional importance for the functioning of the muscular system of the lower extremities during running are the food sources that provide energy for use by these muscles. In prolonged light to moderate running, the muscles use mostly energy that comes from the aerobic metabolism of fat. Under great stress, the muscles switch to the use of carbohydrates in the form of glycogen.

Good marathon runners who function at three-quarters of the maximum capacity remain generally in an aerobic or oxidative state. But if they exceed 80 percent of their maximum capacity, the body switches from the use of fat to glycogen. The resulting depletion of

---

*A high energy phosphate bond that occurs in muscles and supplies them with emergency energy.

muscle glycogen accounts for the severe states of fatigue that occur late in a marathon race. The longer a runner continues to use fat as the main source of metabolism, the longer and harder he or she can run.

MASSAGE

Massage is a great tension reliever; that is, if your masseur knows what he's doing. To know if you're being abused—or to start learning an art that will win you grateful friends—read *The Massage Book* by George Downing.

1. Close your eyes, breathe deeply, relax, and allow the masseur to work without interference. Give your complete attention to the massage and speak only if you're hurt or uncomfortable.
2. Oil (vegetable or mineral) is essential to a good massage because it helps the hands glide over the skin while pressure is being applied. Alcohol can be substituted if nothing else is available.
3. It's best to use a massage table. Working on the floor is possible, but it's more tiring. The masseur should pay attention to how he sits, stands or kneels, and should always keep his back straight.
4. Solitude and quiet are important. Bright lighting should be avoided, and music is a nice touch.
5. Clean hands and short nails are essential. The masseur should always warm both the hands and the oil by rubbing the palms of the hands together before touching the body that is to be massaged.
6. Don't be afraid to apply pressure. The person being massaged will tell you if you're hurting him or her.
7. Maintain even speed and pressure. Change both occasionally, but always gradually.
8. Try not to break contact with the body once the massage is started.
9. Use weight rather than muscles to apply pressure.
10. Concentrate on exploring and defining the underlying structure of the body—feel the tissues and bones and the texture of the muscles.

ALTITUDE TRAINING

Training at high altitudes is a plus! Researchers and altitude-trained athletes have offered the following tips for those who plan to take up altitude training:

1. Most altitude-trained runners live between 5000 and 8000 feet above sea level.
2. Plan to stay in the training area as long as possible. It takes at least a month to adapt. Some of the effects of altitude on running will not become apparent for a year.
3. If you have been training at sea level, cut back on training by as much as 50 percent and gradually increase to your former rate.
4. After three weeks, your body will actually start to change. You will have more oxygen carrying blood cells than before. Each of these cells feeds oxygen to the muscles and helps to keep fatigue away a little longer. You will probably use oxygen more efficiently.
5. Note the increase of myoglobin in the muscle. A subjective sensation of well-being at borderline stress will become evident during the period from four to ten days after returning to your regular training area, and you will notice an ability to maintain a relatively fast pace with a good margin to spare, as well as an ability to mount a long sprint during the final phases of a race.

SPEED INDICATOR

These "test distances" take into account the kind of speed used in the runner's specialty. The half-miler/miler employs the more controlled speed of the 440. The longer-distance runner needs the endurance speed of the mile.

Applying these test distances, we can find a set of speed limits:

880 yards: 440 average five seconds slower than best 440 time
One mile: 440 average ten seconds slower than best 440 time
Two miles: mile average fifteen seconds slower than best mile time
Three miles: mile average twenty seconds slower than best mile time

Six miles: mile average thirty seconds slower than best mile time
Marathon: mile average one minute slower than best mile time

Few runners ever really achieve such low averages. Since endurance
is easier to improve than speed, there's always hope.

PROGRAM PROCEDURES: MARATHON RACE

STAGE 7R: WEEK 1

Day	Workout	Conditions	Comments
1	10 miles		
2	8 miles**		
3	10 miles		
4	18 miles		
5	10 miles*		
6	8 miles		
7	12 miles		

Daily avg.:

Mileage for week:

*See Notes, p. 172.
**See Notes, p. 172.

It's Snowy

Should you wait until it melts even if you have to wait until spring? No! You adapt your running style to the weather conditions and dress and run accordingly. Remember, many an early spring race includes falling or fallen snow.
  If it's hot, think snow!

PROGRAM PROCEDURES: MARATHON RACE

STAGE 7R: WEEK 2

Day	Workout	Conditions	Comments
1	10 miles		
2	8 miles or day off		
3	10 miles*		
4	12 miles		
5	10 miles		
6	8 miles**		
7	18 miles		

Daily avg.:

Mileage for week:

_____

_____

_____

_____

*See Notes, p. 172.
**See Notes, p. 172.

Be sure your racing shoes are carefully broken in—but not overworn—and are ready for action on race day.

You may want to sacrifice lightness for comfort and shock absorption. Light training flats are better than racing flats. Training shoes will make you feel better now. Use racing shoes at races.

PROGRAM PROCEDURES: MARATHON RACE

STAGE 7R: WEEK 3

Day	Workout	Conditions	Comments
1	10 miles		
2	8 miles**		
3	10 miles		
4	12 miles		
5	10 miles* or day off		
6	8 miles		
7	18 miles		

Daily avg.:

Mileage for week:

_____

_____

_____

_____

*See Notes, p. 172.
**See Notes, p. 172.

In cool weather, the body loses heat easily. As the weather becomes warmer, the body must work harder to cool itself. Therefore, sweating becomes more profuse. But sweating, in and of itself, does not accomplish anything other than cooling. It does not help you reduce.

Practice drinking fluids on long runs and races so you'll be used to it on marathon day.

PROGRAM PROCEDURES: MARATHON RACE

STAGE 7R: WEEK 4

Day	Workout	Conditions	Comments
1	10 miles		
2	8 miles**		
3	10 miles		
4	18 miles		
5	10 miles*		
6	8 miles		
7	12 miles (race)		

Daily avg.:

Mileage for week:

*See Notes, p. 172.
**See Notes, p. 172.

To date, the best and cheapest remedy for a cold seems to be moderate amounts of aspirin, liquids, and plenty of rest. You can't sweat it out. There is no evidence that sweating is of any value in removing toxic materials from the body. Nor does sweating promote fitness. Fitness is developed by exercising the muscles of the body.

PROGRAM PROCEDURES: MARATHON RACE

STAGE 7R: WEEK 5

Day	Workout	Conditions	Comments
1	8 miles or day off		
2	10 miles**		
3	14 miles		
4	10 miles		
5	10 miles*		
6	8 miles		
7	20 miles		

Daily avg.:

Mileage for week:

Note: On the long run, time the first half of the run and retrace the distance at a slightly faster tempo. Do not try to race distance or push yourself too hard.
*See Notes, p. 172.
**See Notes, p. 172.

When the snow is high or the pavement is icy or slippery, think twice about running. Many runners are devoted, stubborn people. They hate to give up a day's run for any reason. As the commercial says, they're driven; they must run. They feel sluggish if they don't run. But better a solid sluggishness than a broken bone.

Seek out places that allow for easy foot placement. Try to avoid running on uneven or slippery places.

PROGRAM PROCEDURES: MARATHON RACE

STAGE 7R: WEEK 6

Day	Workout	Conditions	Comments
1	8 miles		
2	10 miles*		
3	14 miles		
4	10 miles or day off		
5	10 miles**		
6	8 miles		
7	20 miles		

Daily avg.:

Mileage for week:

*See Notes, p. 172.
**See Notes, p. 172.

Road salts shorten the life of even the best shoes. The chemicals weaken the fabric of the uppers and can pit the sole materials. Shoes should be rinsed periodically with running water, even those with suede uppers. Be certain that they are thoroughly dry before wearing them again.

PROGRAM PROCEDURES: MARATHON RACE

STAGE 7R: WEEK 7

Day	Workout	Conditions	Comments
1	8 miles		
2	10 miles*		
3	14 miles		
4	10 miles		
5	10 miles**		
6	8 miles		
7	20 miles		

Daily avg.:

Mileage for week:

*See Notes, p. 172.
**See Notes, p. 172.

The skin on your feet tends to dry out when the humidity of the air drops as it cools. If your feet get too dry, they'll crack and bleed. So be sure you keep your feet well oiled with skin lotion to hold in moisture.

PROGRAM PROCEDURES: MARATHON RACE

STAGE 7R: WEEK 8

Day	Workout	Conditions	Comments
1	8 miles or day off		
2	14 miles*		
3	10 miles		
4	20 miles		
5	10 miles**		
6	8 miles		
7	10 miles		

Daily avg.:

Mileage for week:

*See Notes, p. 172.
**See Notes, p. 172.

After heavy training sessions, both superficial and deep massage are very beneficial in relaxing muscle groups and in working out irritated areas. They also improve circulation to the massaged muscles. A biweekly massage, either by a specialist or by a running partner or spouse, can serve as a preventive measure for a runner by relaxing the muscular system and at the same time reducing tension.

PROGRAM PROCEDURES: MARATHON RACE

STAGE 7R: WEEK 9

Day	Workout	Conditions	Comments
1	8 miles		
2	10 miles*		
3	14 miles		
4	10 miles or day off		
5	10 miles**		
6	8 miles		
7	22 miles		

Daily avg.:

Mileage for week:

*See Notes, p. 172.
**See Notes, p. 172.

The key to a successful race lies between the halfway mark and the three-quarter mark. Experienced runners know that if they are in position or on time at the three-quarter mark, the excitement of the finish will usually carry them to the end of the race.

PROGRAM PROCEDURES: MARATHON RACE

STAGE 7R: WEEK 10

Day	Workout	Conditions	Comments
1	8 miles		
2	10 miles*		
3	14 miles		
4	10 miles		
5	10 miles**		
6	8 miles		
7	22 miles		

Daily avg.:

Mileage for week:

_____

_____

_____

*See Notes, p. 172.
**See Notes, p. 172.

Generally speaking, your level of fitness determines the extent to which you can tolerate heat. Those who perspire easily and children are the most vulnerable to heat exhaustion. For the most part, you should run during the cooler times of the day, although some heat training is necessary if you intend to do a great deal of racing between 11:00 A.M. and 2:00 P.M.

Run on race-type terrain. If you are not used to it, a change of terrain can have a drastic effect on your performance in a race.

PROGRAM PROCEDURES: MARATHON RACE

STAGE 7R: WEEK 11

Day	Workout	Conditions	Comments
1	8 miles		
2	10 miles*		
3	14 miles		
4	10 miles**		
5	10 miles		
6	6 miles		
7	10 miles (race)		

Daily avg.:

Mileage for week:

*See Notes, p. 172.
**See Notes, p. 172.

Most runners lose ten pounds in their first year of running without any change in their diet. A half-hour of running will burn 600 calories.

How do you look now?

Fat and protein are slow in getting out of the stomach and into the digestive tract (three to five hours). Athletes must have liquids before an event because they sweat so much.

PROGRAM PROCEDURES: MARATHON RACE

STAGE 7R: WEEK 12

Day	Workout	Conditions	Comments
1	8 miles		
2	18 miles		
3	8 miles		
4	10 miles*		
5	8 miles		
6	10 miles		
7	8 miles**		

Daily avg.:

Mileage for week:

*See Notes, p. 172.
**See Notes, p. 172.

Our workouts are from eight to twenty miles a day (work up to this over a period of months). Usually there are shorter-run days after fast, hard days to allow recovery.

Workouts should be varied as much as possible, but not haphazardly. You must have a plan for success.

Follow a yearly training program that emphasizes endurance training as the key to running development.

PROGRAM PROCEDURES: MARATHON RACE

STAGE 7R: PEAKING WEEK 1

Day	Workout	Conditions	Comments
1	6 miles or day off		
2	7 miles		
3	20 miles		
4	6 miles		
5	9 miles*		
6	6 miles		
7	10 miles		

Daily avg.:

Mileage for week:

*See Notes, p. 172.

Note: The Peaking Week schedules are *not* part of your normal training. You will want to run these programs *only* 2 weeks before a marathon race. It is especially imperative that you concentrate on the quality of your workouts during the peaking stages. Your form should be as close to perfect as possible, and all runs should be performed without stopping to walk. If you can't satisfy those two criteria, you're not ready to try to peak.

A runner without goals is not likely to succeed.

The common denominator of all racing is pain.

Build a positive attitude toward work.

Always have your ditty bag packed and ready to go, so you won't have to run down a long, tedious checklist before every race. Yes, you do *need spare shoelaces and lots and lots of safety pins, and lots of Vaseline.*

PROGRAM PROCEDURES: MARATHON RACE

STAGE 7R: PEAKING WEEK 2

Day	Workout	Conditions	Comments
1	8 miles		
2	13 miles		
3	7 miles		
4	6 miles		
5	6 miles		
6	4 miles		
7	marathon race		

Daily avg.:

Mileage for week:

PROGRAM PROCEDURES: MARATHON RACE

STAGE 7R: RECOVERY WEEK 1

Day	Workout	Conditions	Comments
1	off: soak—Jacuzzi		
2	walk: 20 minutes		
3	jog and walk: 30 minutes		
4	jog and walk: 30 minutes		
5	jog and walk: 40 minutes		
6	jog and walk: 40 minutes		
7	jog and walk: 50 minutes		

Daily avg.:

Mileage for week:

PROGRAM PROCEDURES: MARATHON RACE

STAGE 7R: RECOVERY WEEK 2

Day	Workout	Conditions	Comments
1	5 miles		
2	8 miles		
3	10 miles		
4	6 miles		
5	8 miles		
6	6 miles		
7	12 miles		

Daily avg.:

Mileage for week:

PROGRAM PROCEDURES: MARATHON RACE

STAGE 7R: RECOVERY WEEK 3

Day	Workout	Conditions	Comments
1	6 miles		
2	8 miles		
3	10 miles		
4	6 miles		
5	9 miles		
6	6 miles		
7	14 miles		

Daily avg.: _____

Mileage for week: _____

_____

_____

_____

_____

PROGRAM PROCEDURES: MARATHON RACE

STAGE 7R: RECOVERY WEEK 4

Day	Workout	Conditions	Comments
1	10 miles		
2	8 miles		
3	12 miles		
4	8 miles		
5	10 miles		
6	6 miles		
7	14 miles		

Daily avg.:

Mileage for week:

21

DESIGNING A TRAINING SCHEDULE

The ultimate purpose of a coach is to teach the athlete how to coach himself or herself. We think we have supplied just about every training schedule any hobbyist runner could want. But the day may come when some of you want to design your own training program. Others may be interested in the principles behind this book's training schedules. To help you become the complete runner, we'd like to leave you with an explanation of the theory behind our running program.

You've probably noticed the cyclical nature of our schedules. They take into account a person's natural ability to absorb and adapt to new stress. The training system is based on what we call "stress cycles." The athlete runs one tough workout, then runs easy for 2 or 3 days to recover. Our method works in harmony with the body, instead of trying to subdue or conquer it. The program first establishes basic conditioning, then gradually builds the runner up to greater fitness. In this sytem, the planting and cultivation seasons are long; the harvest comes slowly, but its yield is rich and sure.

Some athletes can achieve equal results with much harder training than is offered in our program. Indeed, some competitive athletes may need such training in order to reach their absolute peak. That can be determined only by an experienced personal coach or by discouraging trial and error. Most people break down under that kind of training, burning out before ever approaching their true potential.

Our slogan is *not* "No Pain, No Gain." That's a stupid approach to athletics. Injuries don't help any runner to improve. Our slogan is "Train, Don't Strain." Be conservative in predicting how much new stress you can take, and build up gradually. This approach makes it inevitable that you will gain more and more strength over the course of your training, and—just as important—that you'll maintain your enthusiasm because you're running without injuries.

As a practical example of our philosophy, you've seen that the week's longest run almost always comes on the last day of the week. It comes when the runner is the most tired; it's the culmination of gradually accumulating loads. The earlier runs have built up the runner's strength, but their immediate effect is to tire him or her. We've programmed in enough of a rest period before this long run to ensure that the normal person will be able to do the long workout. It will just be harder to do on that last day of the training week than it would have been had it come earlier. You've also noticed that the rest periods between harder workouts shorten as you move farther along in the training schedules. Our program builds in intensity not only from day to day, but from week to week. It's exactly the same as the progressive resistance in a Nautilus machine: The farther you go, the more stressful the program becomes. It becomes more stressful because the athlete has been conditioned to handle the stress, and because he or she wants the additional conditioning.

For the competitive racer, these principles apply to anaerobic work as well as to building aerobic endurance. For such an athlete, the distance training serves as a complement to the anaerobic work. The runner's ability to handle increased anaerobic work is a direct result of his or her aerobic base. This fact was long ignored in long-distance running. The results were injured and mentally burned-out long-distance runners.

The anaerobic workouts become gradually more intense as the athlete builds his or her base. The length of speed pick-ups increases, and the rest interval between them shortens. Advanced competitive athletes will run "ladder intervals," where each pick-up is longer than the previous one, and the final one is therefore the longest of all. Because speed pick-ups do no good unless run with good "quality" (speed and form), this very concentrated form of anaerobic training cannot be performed by an athlete who has not

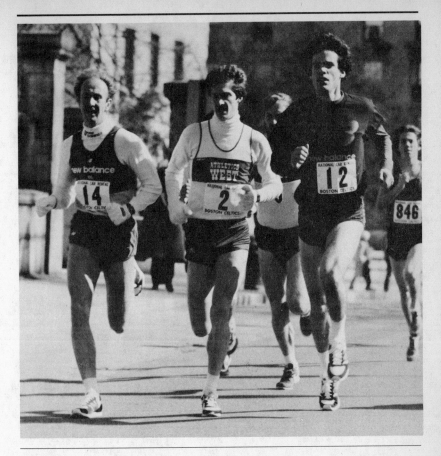

Greg Meyer, Bruce Bickford, and Vin Flemming exhibit top running form in the clutch of competition. (Photograph by Bill Boyle)

been gradually and fully conditioned by easier forms of speedwork. This is an example of what we mean by our program taking a long time to bear fruit, but bearing fruit that is rich and rewarding.

Physiologically, our program embodies the principles discussed in Chapter 2, Body Cycles. Philosophically, the program is characterized by one of Coach Squires's sayings: "Success is that place on the road where preparation and opportunity meet, but too few people recognize it because it comes disguised as sweat and work. Have a good sense of humor, a big dose of patience, and a dash of humility, and you will be rewarded manyfold throughout your running career."

INDEX